"I work in a busy emergency department. Almost every shift I work, I see yet another family in crisis. Children and teens are especially vulnerable to the new and highly potent marijuana products. Laura's tribute to her son and willingness to speak up and out should be applauded. What happened to her son, Johnny, could happen to any child/teen/youth who uses today's high potency marijuana."

Karen Randall, MD, FAAEM
VP Case Management, SCEMA
Certified in Cannabis Science and Medicine,
University of Vermont School of Medicine
Pueblo, CO

"As an enduring tribute to her son, Laura Stack has pulled together an invaluable analysis of the common misconceptions surrounding marijuana which led to his eventual downfall. Marijuana is a large part of the minefield that all teens must navigate in today's world before they reach adulthood, a sobering reality that parents need to see clearly in order to help their children survive and thrive. This book provides a solid framework to assist in that process while making ample use of references to the best and most relevant scientific literature out there."

Christine L. Miller, PhD
Neuroscientist
MillerBio
Baltimore, Maryland

"Laura and John Stack are brave enough to write about the loss of their son, Johnny. This is something every parent should read, whether or not they know of a young person battling issues related to today's dangerous marijuana. Please share Johnny's message."

Kenneth Finn, MD
Springs Rehabilitation, PC
Volunteer Clinical Instructor at the University
of Colorado Medical School, Colorado Springs Branch
Colorado Springs, CO

D1595822

"Laura Stack has constructed a beautiful legacy for her son, allowing Johnny's story to help guide the actions and decisions of other teenagers and families. Laura has long had an unmistakable passion and gift for writing; it's no mistake that she has created such a seamless blend of personal narrative and empirical science. If you do your family the favor of reading this book, you'll come away with all the tools and information you'll need to protect your children from the ever-increasing social pressures of marijuana normalization. Your time could not be better spent."

Aaron Weiner, PhD, ABPP
Licensed Clinical Psychologist
Board-Certified in Counseling Psychology (ABPP)
Master Addiction Counselor (MAC)
Lake Forest, IL

"Thank you to Laura Stack for her courage to share her family's story. Today's marijuana may be packaged as medicine but can be deadly poison for teenagers. The developing brain is one of the world's greatest resources. So, the message in this book is crucial to disseminate."

Christian Thurstone, MD
Child and Addiction Psychiatrist
Professor of Psychiatry at the University of
Colorado School of Medicine
Denver, CO

"This is a remarkable book with a powerful message for parents about the devastating and unpredictable negative consequences of marijuana use for some youth. It is also a passionate story of the painful struggles families often have trying to help youth who are addicted to marijuana and other drugs. A wake-up call in the face of widespread denial of the serious adverse consequences many people suffer from marijuana use, this book sends a powerful message to parents about the importance of helping youth grow into adulthood drug-free because of the unique vulnerability of the adolescent brain to the chemical seduction of drug use."

Robert L. DuPont, MD
President, Institute for Behavior and Health, Inc.
First Director, National Institute on Drug Abuse;
Second White House Drug Chief

"I am full of admiration for Laura Stack who has turned the tragedy of her son's death into a mission to educate other parents about the harms associated with cannabis use. We need parents to tell their stories. It is the most powerful testimony. Laura Stack has created a beautiful legacy for her son Johnny and has given parents a voice in this sad, yet ultimately hopeful book written in his memory."

Mary Cannon
Professor of Psychiatric Epidemiology and Youth Mental Health
RCSI University of Medicine and Health Sciences
Dublin, Ireland

"Laura and John's brave account of their son's devastating tragedy serves as a warning sign and a critical call to action for all who love and care for young people. Their story illustrates how the foe we face rides on the wheels of capitalism and runs over our children. When regulation and consumer protection are absent, we need ambassadors to arm our children with neurodevelopmental science and empower parents' voices. Thank you, Laura, for sharing your story and for starting Johnny's Ambassadors."

Crystal Collier, PhD, LPC-S
Therapist, Researcher, Educator,
BrainAbouts Prevention Program Creator & Director
Houston, Texas

"Laura Stack has been able to turn a tragedy no parent should ever have to experience into something so powerful and helpful to all people who may be struggling with the normalization of very potent versions of marijuana that is no longer the healing plant many people thought it was. The messages in this book are important and so needed at this time to help protect generations to come from the devastating impacts of high potency THC marijuana."

Libby Stuyt, MD
Addiction Psychiatrist
Colorado

"This is a powerful book for everyone; parents, grandparents, and young people should read it. Written from the heart of a mother, Laura Stack, who has transformed her immense pain from losing a son into something extremely valuable for everyone. The message is clear: strong cannabis risks mental well-being and can even lead to fatality, as it sadly did in her son Johnny's case."

Zerrin Atakan, MD
Senior Cannabis Researcher
King's College
London, UK

"I wish I could say that this is the first time I have read or heard the story of a bright, happy, gifted child and beloved son's downwards spiral into depression, psychosis, despair, and suicide after becoming addicted to cannabis. As a researcher and clinician who has been treating adolescents with substance and mental health problems for nearly 30 years, it is not the first time. I would strongly urge clinicians and parents to read this book with the hope that together, we can make Johnny's story uncommonly rare."

Paula Riggs, MD, Professor
Director, Division of Addiction Science, Prevention & Treatment
Vice Chair, Faculty Affairs, Department of Psychiatry
University of Colorado School of Medicine

"Laura Stack is a new and powerful voice on this important subject. She is knowledgeable, passionate, and sensible—a rare combination in this space. Laura has taken the time to be educated, and she is using what she knows to impact lives. While many will focus on the tragedy of her story, I see her words and actions as a beacon of light, shining to help others find their way through the dark. Laura and her family's true legacy is sharing Johnny's story to keep them from following his path."

Ben Cort
CEO, the Foundry
Author, Weed, Inc.
Steamboat Springs, CO

"Laura Stack has transformed the tragic death of her son into a positive movement and narrative to alert parents, youth, and policy makers on the hazards of marijuana and its lamentable outcomes in vulnerable users. Her compelling book proffers the grief of her son's story combined with objective information that should be digested by those who believe that marijuana is a safe, non-addictive drug. We revere the human brain and aspire to protect it from drug-induced injuries, compromised function, and disease. Why? From my perspective and many on the front lines of public health, medicine, or neurobiology, this is not a war on drugs, but instead, a defense of our brains—the repository of our humanity."

Bertha K. Madras, PhD
Professor of Psychobiology, Department of Psychiatry
Harvard Medical School and McLean Hospital
Belmont, MA

the dangerous TRUTH about today's MARIJUANA

JOHNNY STACK'S LIFE & DEATH STORY

LAURA STACK

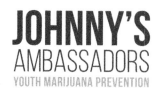

JOHNNY'S
AMBASSADORS
YOUTH MARIJUANA PREVENTION

Published by Johnny's Ambassadors Publishing.
9948 Cottoncreek Drive, Highlands Ranch, CO 80130
www.JohnnysAmbassadors.org

ISBN 979-8-9873481-0-9

Printed in the United States of America.

DEDICATION

To Johnny

I promise.

CONTENTS

FOREWORD

By Kevin Sabet

Having become a parent for the first time in 2019, my little girl is now my whole world. I cannot fathom what Laura and John must have gone through on November 20, 2019. While I was at home getting to know my then two-week-old, Laura and John were going through unimaginable anguish.

That is why what the Stacks have done to honor Johnny in a short year with Johnny's Ambassadors is nothing short of extraordinary. Determined to teach all of America her son's name, Laura—a force of nature—has transformed her grief into action in her home state of Colorado and across the country and indeed, the world.

And action we need. Badly.

Since the Mile High State took its nickname quite literally in 2012—as a result of a multimillion-dollar financed referendum based primarily on untruths—the state has suffered. In Colorado, pot retail locations outnumber all McDonald's and Starbucks locations combined—promoting a culture of normalization.

And this has had consequences: In Colorado, the number of marijuana-related emergency department visits increased 54 percent from 2013 to 2017, according to the state health department. Yearly marijuana-related hospitalizations increased 101 percent in that same period. Calls to the poison control center for marijuana exposures also increased. In 2013, 125 calls were made for marijuana-related exposures. By 2018, that number jumped to 266, representing a 112.8 percent increase. Youth cases (instances of marijuana-related exposures of children aged eight or younger) increased 126.2 percent from 2013 to 2018. In 2018, youth cases represented over half of all marijuana-related exposure calls. All of this translates into money spent, yes, but also into lives ruined.

To add insult to injury, we know this is affecting small children, not just older teens. A study by the Colorado Department of Public Health and Environment found that in 2018, over 23,000 homes in the state with children aged one to 14 years had marijuana products stored unsafely. In 2018, 60 percent of youth marijuana exposures involved edibles, compared with just 18 percent in 2016. Even when packaging is compliant with Colorado's regulatory requirements, it fails to discourage or prevent children from accessing potent and dangerous marijuana.

Childproof packaging and warning labels don't seem to be helping. The state's Regional Center for Poison Control and Prevention (RPC) recorded a 140 percent increase in marijuana exposures, and the drug was cited in 23 percent of Colorado school suspensions, the highest of all documented school offenses. Further, between 2012 and 2014, the percentage of 10- to 14-year-olds who once or twice tested positive for THC increased from 19 percent to 23 percent; those who tested positive three or more times increased from 18 percent to 25 percent. There are countless other statistics about increasing numbers of car crashes related to THC intoxication, workplace dangers, and targeting of vulnerable and minority communities in the state.

But I am hopeful for the future. Because of advocacy from Laura and other like-minded groups, decision makers—for the first time—are now contemplating a limit on the amount of THC that can be sold in the state. Capping potency rates would be a much-needed game-changer that would save lives.

This doesn't mean users should be jailed. While we should remove criminal penalties for use, expunge records, and invest in prevention and treatment, the legalization of marijuana has become akin to mass commercialization, or as I like to say, addiction for profit. Scientific literature on the harms of marijuana use exists in abundance. According to the National Academies of Sciences, there are over 20,000 peer-reviewed research articles linking marijuana use to severe mental health outcomes ranging from depression to psychosis, as well as consequences for physical health and brain development, among other risks. These are often lost in conversations about legalization.

Also lost is the role of a new, commercialized industry that makes money off heavy users. Like the alcohol and tobacco industries, marijuana makes most of its money from the one in four users who consume more than 80 percent of the product, according to a state of Colorado study. The industry, then, has an incentive to promote heavy use. This is not about "casual" marijuana smoking by the otherwise non-using adult. This is about garnering lifelong customers and starting them young. Remember Joe Camel?

No one knows what the 2020s will bring in terms of pot policy. One thing for sure is that the Mad Men of Marijuana will continue to work hard to addict you and your kids. We've been tricked by other industries before. You know the saying, "Fool me once, shame on you. Fool me twice, shame on me."

Laura and Johnny's Ambassadors will help all of us navigate these tricky waters and ensure none of us are fooled, no matter what policies get passed in DC or our state capitals. After all, parents have more influence on a child's decision to use—to do anything, really—than anyone else, including more than siblings, peers, teachers, or celebrities. I think we parents sometimes underestimate this awesome responsibility. We think, *Why would my child listen to me?* The truth is, they do.

Laura, through her powerful, moving, timely journey, can teach us all quite a lot. This book is a treasure.

Kevin A. Sabet, Ph.D.
President, Smart Approaches to Marijuana (SAM)
Author, *Smokescreen: What the Marijuana Industry Doesn't Want You to Know*

INTRODUCTION

My cell phone rang at 1:03 a.m., on Thursday, November 21, 2019, and I woke with a start. I always kept my ringtone volume on full blast so I would be sure to awaken to Johnny's late-night calls. I reached over to pick up the phone, fully expecting to see Johnny's name on the screen. Instead, it said Douglas County Sheriff's Office.

"Hello?"

"Hello, Ma'am, I'm with the Douglas County Sheriff's Office. I'm at your front door. Will you please come down and let us in?"

"Do you have Johnny with you?"

"No, Ma'am. I'm sorry…I do not."

A cold chill slithered through my veins. I rolled over and shook John's shoulder. "John, wake up. The police are at the door. It's Johnny again."

My husband jumped out of bed. We threw on our robes and hurried downstairs. John yanked open the door. A uniformed police officer stood there with a woman in a black shirt and pants. We motioned for them to come inside and led them into the living room.

Almost instinctively, John and I sat down on the sofa. "What happened?"

The woman in black said, "Mr. and Mrs. Stack, I'm with the coroner's office. I'm so sorry to tell you that your son is deceased."

I stared at her for a few seconds. "Deceased? What do you mean—deceased?"

"He's dead, Ma'am...he jumped off the roof of the RTD parking garage on Park Meadows Drive."

I heard myself screaming as I fell into John's arms. And for the next few moments, I heard nothing.

Every parent's worst nightmare. I was now living it, breathing it, suffocating in it. Even as I heard myself wail, the conversation of only three days ago flashed into my mind. Looking back, Johnny had warned us over dinner.

"Mom, I just want you to know you were right. You were right all along. You told me marijuana would hurt my brain. Marijuana has ruined my mind and my life. I'm sorry, and I love you."

This is the life-and-death story of our beloved, forever 19-year-old son, Johnny.

CHAPTER 1:
THE BELOVED SON

February 7, 2000 —
Raising Johnny by Laura

To introduce myself, Johnny's mother, I grew up in Colorado Springs, Colorado, on the grounds of the United States Air Force Academy (USAFA). My father was a colonel, had a Ph.D., and taught ethics and philosophy to the cadets. My mother was a psychologist and lecturer, and she provided Christian counseling services. They could both talk non-stop for weeks about their areas of expertise. Education, writing, and oratory were all important to them. It's not surprising I became a professional speaker and have authored books on the topics of productivity and performance. Now I'm the Founder & CEO of Johnny's Ambassadors, the 501(c)(3) nonprofit we established after Johnny's death (*JohnnysAmbassadors.org*).

I had a lovely childhood, protected in many ways from the outside world. As you'd expect, I grew up with a lot of structure and discipline. I was raised in the Catholic church. I was outgoing and participated in student council, cheerleading, dance, and theater. I enjoyed schoolwork and focused heavily on my grades.

In high school in the mid-80s, a friend managed to get some weed. Usually, we were lucky if we could find some 3.2 beer and sneak down to the "beer tree." We had to be sneaky, because if the police—or heaven forbid, our parents caught us with weed—we would all be in huge trouble. We all tried it since we wanted to know what it was like to get high. I didn't like it at all; it made my head spin. My friends thought it would be funny to shine a strobe light in my eyes, and I became very dizzy. So basically, it wasn't a good experience.

Tetrahydrocannabinol (THC) is the chemical in marijuana that makes you high. Back then, our "grass" contained a very low level of THC, about 2-4%. Today's flower can be over 40% THC, and THC concentrates can be 90+% THC. Today's narcotic-strength marijuana makes it a hard drug in a new class all on its own, as we'll soon discuss in the research.

Admittedly, I didn't know anything had changed since I was in high school because I haven't used marijuana since then. Adolescent concentrate usage wasn't even tracked by the Colorado Department of Public Health and Environment (CDPHE) until 2015. New-fangled, high-potency THC concentrates hit the market, and very quietly, marijuana changed. So, my experience with marijuana from high school was my perception going into parenthood. I just didn't know. But I desperately want YOU to know.

Today's teens perceive a lower level of risk if they get caught because it seems more acceptable since it's legal. But teens are at a much greater risk due to the higher level of potency. I'm writing this book for all the parents and grandparents who also smoked marijuana in their younger days and think, "Ah, what's the big deal? It's just pot. I did it too, and I turned out fine." The media and Big Pot also target our youth with marketing messages, assuring them it's medicinal, safe, natural, and legal. Of course, they need to addict their next generation of users, so the pot industry will not acknowledge the significant risks nor will they take responsibility for illegal use by our children. In turn, children tell their parents, "Everyone does it—it's legal—it's natural—it's harmless."

Nothing could be further from the truth. According to Dr. Christian Thurstone, Director of Behavioral Health at Denver Health, a professor of psychiatry at the University of Colorado School of Medicine and a member of Johnny's Ambassadors Scientific Advisory Board, *no level of marijuana use is safe for children*. Why? Because their brains continue to develop into their mid-20s (for girls) and late-20s (for boys).

Here are some things you should know about my beliefs:

- I don't believe people should go to jail for having some marijuana in their pockets.
- I am personally against the legalization of marijuana at any level and wouldn't vote for it; however, I believe Americans use the ballot box to make controversial decisions.
- Where marijuana is legal, we need to put better guardrails in place and tighten regulatory loopholes to protect our youth.
- I believe if you can't get alcohol and cigarettes until 21 years of age, you shouldn't be able to get "medical" marijuana either.
- Marijuana can harm anyone at any age; however, adolescents, teens, and young adults are particularly vulnerable. At

Johnny's Ambassadors, we work hard to educate youth and parents as a primary prevention strategy.

Even pro-marijuana adults have told me they don't want kids using marijuana recreationally, so we can focus on *that* area of agreement.

Now to tell you about Johnny.

John Kenneth Stack was born in Highlands Ranch, Colorado, on February 7, 2000, at 9:19 a.m., and died on November 20, 2019, in Lone Tree, Colorado, at 10:32 p.m. Since he was born in early 2000, you'll be able to conveniently determine his age throughout this book. We called him Johnny to avoid confusion between him and my husband, who is also named John.

Johnny was a sweet, intelligent, happy, and handsome child. He was funny, sensitive, and creative. When he was a young boy, I constantly laughed at his antics. He was his momma's boy, and I was "his person."

Every night, he wanted me to read with him, pray with him, and sing lullabies while rubbing his back as he fell asleep. He had a favorite blanket and a little well-loved white-and-gray stuffed animal named Wolfie. He loved going to the zoo, collecting bugs, and petting dogs on all our walks. His favorite food was pizza, and his favorite treat was Krispy Kreme doughnuts. Even when he was 11 years old, I was still rubbing his back while praying and singing with him.

Johnny loved the ocean, video games, books, Legos, computers, math, and music (especially Billy Joel). In his lifetime, he participated in baseball, swimming, archery, soccer, basketball, cross country, track, karate, and guitar and piano lessons. He loved going to summer camps and even agreed to go to Cotillion to learn how to dance.

He had a spirit of service, a beautiful smile, and a kind heart. Johnny was highly intelligent, both intellectually and emotionally. Until he got sick, he was a loyal friend and a loving son. He was on the honor roll every semester, had a 4.0 GPA, and earned a scholarship to Colorado State University.

Johnny loved to travel. When I traveled to my speaking engagements, I would often pull one of the three kids out of school to spend private time together. Johnny and I enjoyed a memorable trip to Kansas City, where he ate his first huge Tomahawk steak, BBQ ribs, and pan-fried chicken. Johnny's favorite place in all the world was Hawaii. Each year, we would treat our family to a trip to one of the islands, using the mileage points I'd collected from traveling the previous year. Johnny and I used to feed the stray cats at the hotels. When we arrived, we would go to the grocery store and buy canned cat food. We would wander around finding cats and then leave food for them under the bushes or wherever they lived. Random, I know, but we enjoyed it.

Johnny really enjoyed history. He was interested in world history in general but especially American and Greek history. One year, our oldest child, Meagan, went to Exeter, England, for an international semester with Colorado State University. Because of the way the semesters were scheduled, she wouldn't return home until January, after Christmas. So, our whole family traveled to London and spent Christmas with her. Johnny and I especially loved the museums! Our favorite collection of medieval weapons and armor was in the Tower of London. Our poor family had to practically drag us out of there because Johnny and I hung out for hours, reading every single card in the displays.

Johnny and I liked to find ugly fruits and vegetables. Every time we went into a grocery store anywhere, we would find a weird-looking item. We would look it up online, figure out how to cook it or otherwise prepare it, and eat it together. We had big laughs over how some of them tasted as bad as they looked.

I could spend the entire book telling you all about who he was before the marijuana; instead, I invite you to watch a six-minute video review of his life at *JohnnysAmbassadors.org/tribute*. Two dear friends, Brian Walter and Sylvie Di Giusto, created this tribute for me to show at his memorial service. Through pictures and videos, you'll gain a sense of what a wonderful person he was and get to know him a little since you likely didn't meet him.

You'll see that we are a regular suburban family and did regular family things. Johnny had a happy life and a family who loved him very much. Unfortunately, we live in Colorado which was the first state to legalize recreational marijuana in 2012. It became available in 2014 when Johnny was 14 years old.

February 7, 2000 — John's 2019 Eulogy: Raising Johnny

Dear family and friends, thank you for coming today. You honor Johnny and our whole family by being here.

We are here to celebrate the life of Johnny Stack and to say goodbye to a beloved son and wonderful person.

I'm Johnny's father, also John Stack. Johnny was the fifth John in the Stack family line. We all had different middle names, so we didn't have to have a junior. My wife Laura and I are also parents to Meagan and James, and you will also hear from them today.

Laura and I named Johnny in honor of our fathers. Johnny was named John Kenneth for my father John, and Laura's father Kenneth. Johnny and his grandfather John became close when my dad had lived with us for a year and a half during his battle with cancer. He lost that battle in 2017, and we like to think that Dad was one of the first to welcome Johnny into heaven. They share a niche outside in the memorial garden, and we invite you to stop by following the service.

During this short time, I'd like to share some of my favorite memories about Johnny.

Johnny loved amusement parks. I remember Johnny being just tall enough by his hair sticking up to ride the fastest roller coaster at Six Flags. He was jump-up-and-down excited. As we exited the coaster, he said, "Let's go again!" And we did—repeatedly.

When he was around ten, we took a trip to Universal Studios in Orlando. Johnny, James, and I went to the park early before the ladies. We ran to be first on the twin coasters that race each other, which was then called the Dragon Challenge. As we exited the coaster, we discovered a secret shortcut to get back in line. So, we just kept going back on the ride, over and over again, maybe five or six times. I finally said, "I've had enough!" So, the boys let me sit it out, and they rode together another three or four times before they finally came off.

One of the things that I loved about Johnny was his sense of humor. I loved hearing him laugh, and he made us laugh. Our family had an Easter tradition that was passed down from my wife's father, Ken. After all the baskets and plastic eggs were found, the children would gather around me in the kitchen. Laura would take out the basket of hard-boiled eggs that were colored the day before, and each child would take a turn cracking an egg on my head. I always thought at some point the kids would outgrow this tradition, but it still lives on to this day. Last year, my son James went first, and he cracked me just a little too hard for my liking. I said, "Wow, that was a bit rough! Can we dial this back a few notches?" Next up was Johnny, and he said, "Don't worry, Dad!" He very gently cracked his egg, and it quickly became apparent something wasn't quite right. While James distracted me, Johnny had switched his egg with a raw one from the fridge, and it was now squishing down the side of my head. Johnny thought that was funny, and so did everyone else. Except me.

Johnny loved the ocean. We could spend hours at the beach running into the waves, playing in the sand, or tossing a football. One special memory is the time we went snorkeling in Hanauma Bay on Oahu in Hawaii. We floated around for hours and saw countless varieties of fish. A few days before he died, Johnny talked about taking his new dog, Benji, to show him the ocean.

So, when we were discussing Johnny's cremation, we knew right away that we wanted to keep some of Johnny's ashes separate. They are in a special urn we will take to Hawaii and scatter the ashes in the ocean in a place he loved so much.

I loved my son, and I miss him. But I am encouraged by God's holy word. Philippians 3:21 says, "Who, by the power that enables Him to bring everything under His control, will transform our lowly bodies so that they will be like His glorious body." We take comfort in knowing that God has the power to transform our bodies and keep us secure with Him. I truly believe God has Johnny, and we will see him again in heaven.

February 7, 2000 — James' 2019 Eulogy: Growing Up with Johnny

I'm James. I'm Johnny's brother. I have a lot of wonderful memories of my older brother and best friend and just wanted to share a few of those with you today.

I remember going on vacation with Johnny, and we would always argue over who was going to have to sleep on the couch and who had the bed. We would typically decide who got first pick by playing best out of seven games of rock-paper-scissors. Each game was more intense than the last.

We played a lot of video games together across the hall in our separate bedrooms, either alone or with his friends. He was consistently better than everyone else, so we got into a lot of spats because he usually beat me. Believe it or not, I actually miss those arguments with him. After we pretended to go to bed, we would get up again after Mom and Dad went to bed and keep playing.

Since Johnny and I were so close in age—16 months—my mom enrolled both of us in the same activities, so I always had a built-in buddy. From swim lessons to summer camps, from karate to hanging out on vacations, we were inseparable growing up. Just being with him and hanging out are big parts of my childhood memories with him. I miss that. As we got older, our interests shifted, so we didn't spend as much time together, but we were always close.

My brother was so much smarter than I am. I mean, he was a genius. I always looked up to him in school since he was a year older than me, so naturally, I was worried I wouldn't be able to accomplish what he did. When I struggled with calculus, however, and don't tell my mom, he did my homework for me.

We weren't perfect siblings, but no one really is, and I loved him.

February 7, 2000 — Meagan's 2019 Eulogy: Growing Up with Johnny

I'm Meagan, Johnny's older sister. I loved being a family of five. I loved squeezing the five of us into one car, fighting as we got older about who got stuck with the middle seat. For some strange reason, I lost more and more of those fights as the boys grew older and bigger. But as their older sister, I loved watching Johnny and James grow up together, just 16 months apart. From their matching outfit days to the hours spent playing video games together in separate bedrooms, which I will never understand, my younger brothers brought a joy and pride to my life unlike any other.

In every moment of Johnny's precious life, there was a strength in this family that constantly left me in awe. Life with Johnny wasn't always the easiest, but it was always filled with love. Johnny's life taught me that mental health is not a choice. But love is a choice. Love is always present, even when it's not apparent. And I rest easy, knowing how much Johnny loved us and knowing how much he knew he was loved.

Every year, Mom would drag us out for our family photos. When we were younger, we would drive to the Toys-R-Us down the street and awkwardly cram into new poses every year until we ran out of room on that tiny ledge. Finally, for all our sanity, I convinced her to move our photos to outdoor locations, and we went to Lake Dillon, Breckenridge, the Highlands Ranch Mansion, and most recently, right in our own backyard at Daniels Gate. What I treasure most about these photos each year aren't the photos themselves; it's the moments of connection I felt with the boys, rolling our eyes at the silliness of it all, but doing it anyway because we understood how much it meant to Mom.

Mom, the memories I have of the last few years of family photos are some of my favorite moments with Johnny (and honestly, some of the best selfies we've ever taken). Thank you for forcing those family photos on us all these years.

Beyond the photos were plenty of other memorable moments with Johnny taking the starring role. From getting bitten by the parrot after being told not to get too close, to causing an emergency stop on the road to Hana after a bit too much candy and one too many curves in the road, Johnny always kept us on our toes. I remember hours of playing Concentration around the campfire, always amazed and slightly jealous of Johnny's ability to consistently beat us all.

Johnny was by far the smartest of the three of us kids. I remember hours upon hours of him explaining his complex thoughts and innovations that I could never fully understand. All his ideas were rooted in his desire to make a difference in this world and help the people around him. One of my last experiences with Johnny sums up the heart he had for others. He was driving out to see my new house for the first time, and in typical Johnny fashion, he was running late. When he arrived almost an hour late, I asked him what had taken him so long. Apparently, he had found a homeless man freezing on the side of the road and offered to drive him to a homeless shelter 20 minutes away to get out of the cold. Even after their arrival at the shelter, Johnny stayed with him in line until his housing was arranged before leaving to drive over to my place.

Johnny didn't always know how to help himself, yet he always found ways to help those around him. I will never fully understand my brother or many of the choices he made, but I'm proud of the man he was striving to be. And even though it hurts, I'm so thankful for the time we had with him and all the love, joy, and strength his life brought to our family. Thank you all for being here today to celebrate his life and support us during this time.

If you are struggling, please find the courage to reach out — you are loved, you are cherished, and you will be missed far more than you can ever imagine. Thank you.

May 10, 2009 — Mother's Day Poem by Johnny

Ten Things I Like About My Mother

1) When I am sad, she always tries to cheer me up and comfort me.

2) If I don't understand something on my homework, she explains it to me.

3) My mom loves me more than anyone (except James, Dad, and Meagan).

4) She likes to play Go Fish with me and my family.

5) My mom wants me to be safe. She says look both ways before crossing the street.

6) Every day after school, she asks me how my day was, and I tell her.

7) My mom is funny and has a great sense of humor.

8) She loves wildlife and going camping with our family.

9) She is a speaker and has won many rewards speaking.

10) My mom is a terrific parent and is very nice.

Happy Mother's Day 2009!

Love,

Johnny

January 10, 2010 — Baptism

Johnny was baptized *again* today. I used to think, "My kids would never be drug addicts because we raised them in the church, so they have a solid value system." To be sure, your child's faith is a protective factor, but it's not a guarantee he or she won't become a drug addict. Johnny was baptized as an infant at Cherry Hills Community Church in Highlands Ranch, Colorado. Then he prayed with John when he was a young boy and asked Jesus into his heart. He voluntarily asked to be baptized again when he was almost 10 years old.

Johnny was an active participant in the church, not passive. He sang in the kids' choir as a young boy. He attended youth group at church every week, even into high school. He participated in the Awana and Bible Blast programs for many years, winning many trophies and awards for scripture memorization. He enjoyed attending Christian summer camps such as Super Kids Sports Camp at our church, Hume Lake in San Diego, and Idrahaje and Camp Timberline in the mountains. Johnny loved to help other people, particularly the homeless and underprivileged. We volunteered as a family to teach Sunday School for preschoolers for many years, cleaned up the community for our church's Love in Action Day, and delivered Thanksgiving meals to the less fortunate.

Raising your child to be a person of religious faith is a protective factor to be sure. But being a Godly person with great values will not keep your child from becoming addicted to marijuana. Johnny was still human and gave into human temptations, but that wasn't a reflection on how much he loved the Lord.

CHAPTER 2:
THE TEENAGE YEARS

Bottom line, Johnny was a happy boy with a happy life. So, let's fast forward to Johnny's teenage years which is why you are reading this book, I'm guessing.

After Johnny died, I became obsessed with finding out if something had happened to him beyond the marijuana use. I asked his friends from childhood, high school, and college. I secured doctor, psychiatrist, and mental hospital records. I had an in-person visit with his therapist, John Davis, to ask if Johnny had ever revealed anything about being traumatized or sexually abused as a child. Nothing. He was not psychotic or depressed before he used marijuana.

I was getting a lot of questions about Johnny's mental state and whether he was using marijuana to self-medicate a mental illness, a common tactic of many pro-marijuana folks who try blaming a pre-existing condition. So, given the questions I was being asked, there were two issues I investigated around medication and genetic mental illness.

First, Johnny's cheeks would flush when he was embarrassed. Like many teenagers, Johnny was nervous about giving presentations in front of his classmates because he was nervous about turning red. This happened to my other children, too, so I reassured him that *most* people hate talking in front of a group of people. We tried lotions and laser treatments, but nothing seemed to help the flushing. His dislike of public speaking increased after he started using marijuana (more about that coming up). I suspect it was because he became increasingly paranoid about people watching him in general. So, when he was a junior in high school, I took him to his primary care doctor who prescribed a medication called Metoprolol, a beta-blocker to treat high blood pressure. Taking one before a presentation would keep his heart from racing.

After Johnny died, I wondered if the Metoprolol could have contributed, so I researched it and talked to doctors. On rare occasions, Metoprolol has been reported to cause visual hallucinations in the elderly. Johnny never reported hallucinations of any type, auditory or visual, and he took it infrequently. He was young and healthy, and his marijuana use preceded that medication. So, I was satisfied when I was told the medication wasn't a factor.

Second, I investigated the possibility of a genetic predisposition to mental illness from Johnny's grandfather, John Drew, which is an important possibility to understand. When I met my husband, John (James), he told me his parents had divorced when John was eleven years old which made his dad 44 years old at the time. He moved into a house by himself, never worked or drove again, and lived on Supplemental Security Income (SSI). He rode his bicycle to the store and didn't participate in social activities. John never knew why as he was too young.

When I first met Dad, he was nervous about having company in his house but was sweet and quiet. He was indeed a bit odd, but I couldn't put my finger on it. For example, he had a habit of keeping a list of everything he did and the time he did it which seemed a bit like Obsessive Compulsive Disorder to me. Johnny had always been meticulous as well. He was the only one of my three kids whose bedroom was clean, and he didn't like germs.

John's dad lived in Washington, Pennsylvania, where John grew up, until he developed prostate cancer in 2014. When Johnny was 14 years old, he came to live with us in Colorado so we could take care of him. Sweet and quiet, he still wrote timed activities in his little notebook. He mostly kept to himself in his bedroom, watched television, and emerged for meals. He had an odd habit of hiding from me. He would crack his bedroom door on the main level, peek out to see if I was in the kitchen, and then quickly run across the hall to the restroom. "I see you, Dad!" I would call out from the kitchen and laugh.

After a year and a half, his cancer improved enough that he was able to move out of our home and into a condo we own a couple miles away. Oh, how he loved that condo! It was the same one Johnny would live in until he died. Dad lived another year and a half before passing away from the cancer.

After Johnny died, I wanted to understand more about his grandfather's mental condition, so I questioned John's mother (Johnny's grandmother), who is now 81. Understandably, she didn't remember much from 50 years before. She said he had a "social problem" and that he "couldn't be in relationships." She described what seemed like a type of reclusive disorder. He didn't take medication but simply lived alone when they divorced.

So, I did a lot of research on personality disorders. Dad seemed to fit the profile of schizoid personality disorder (or SPD) which is an uncommon condition in which people avoid social activities and consistently shy away from interaction with others. It is often characterized by a tendency toward a solitary or sheltered lifestyle, secretiveness, emotional coldness, detachment, and apathy. This sounded like Dad but didn't resemble Johnny at all.

According to the *Diagnostic and Statistical Manual of Mental Disorders (DSM-5)*, a personality disorder can be diagnosed if there are significant impairments in self and interpersonal functioning together with one or more pathological personality traits. The DSM-5 lists ten personality disorders and allocates each to one of three groups or "clusters": A, B, or C. Cluster A is described as odd, bizarre, and eccentric. SPD falls into this category, and Dad certainly was odd.

In addition, these features must be (1) relatively stable across time and consistent across situations, (2) not better understood as normative for the individual's developmental stage or socio-cultural environment, and (3) not solely due to the direct effects of a substance or general medical condition. Dad was stable across time with his condition. He wasn't in a developmental stage, and he wasn't under the influence of substances. The onset of SPD is in early adulthood, and this happened when Dad was much older, so it's impossible to know for sure if that's what he had. Who's to say Dad had a "significant disorder" versus a convenient label for someone with extreme social anxiety? He was never anything but kind to me and told me he loved me every day.

In contrast, Johnny's psychiatrist said he had straight psychosis with delusional thinking which is typical of mental disorders such as schizoaffective disorder, bipolar, and schizophrenia, not a personality disorder. WebMD.com defines psychosis as "a condition that affects the way your brain processes information. It causes you to lose touch with reality. You might see, hear, or believe things that aren't real. Psychosis is a symptom, not an illness. A mental or physical illness, substance abuse, or extreme stress or trauma can cause it."

While personality disorders may differ from mental disorders, they both lead to significant impairment. After reading this story of John's father, some pro-marijuana folks will say, "Ah! See there, that proves it—Johnny was pre-disposed to mental illness!" Perhaps Johnny inherited some of the cluster of genes from his grandfather that would have led to a mental disorder, regardless of whether he smoked marijuana or not.

I continued to do my research and reached out to experts. I will be quoting Christine Miller, Ph.D., frequently in this book, so I want to thank her for her time and caring. She has been instrumental in helping me understand much of the complex research around marijuana, psychosis, and suicide. Dr. Miller is a graduate of the University of Colorado Health Sciences Center. She earned her Ph.D. in Pharmacology through the Neuroscience Training Program. Her professional history includes both instructor and research associate at Johns Hopkins School of Medicine, postdoctoral fellow at Mental Health Research Institute and Johns Hopkins School of Medicine, and research microbiologist at U.S. Geological Survey. Dr. Miller has been published in peer-reviewed journals more than 30 times in her 30-year career. Currently, Dr. Miller is the president and founder of MillerBio, a firm dedicated to behavioral pharmacology research and consulting. Her areas of research include genetic loci associated with risk for psychosis, the biochemical basis for major mental disorders, biomarkers of psychiatric state and suicidality, and animal models of pharmacotherapy.

She wrote in "The Impact of Marijuana on Mental Health" in *Contemporary Health Issues on Marijuana* (K. Winters and K. Sabet, eds.) Oxford University Press:

> Even in those with a heavy family history of schizophrenia, for example those with an identical twin who is diagnosed with schizophrenia, only about half the time will the other twin develop schizophrenia as well (reviewed by Gottesman & Shields, 1967, and as is evident in the data of Shakoor et al., 2015). The genetic "penetrance" of this disease is far from complete. Thus, the impact of marijuana in an individual with high genetic risk for schizophrenia has both consequence and meaning because no one is destined to develop schizophrenia as a result of their genetic makeup alone. Even should the majority of those at risk prove to be those with a positive family history of psychosis in either 1st- or 2nd-degree relatives, at least 10% of the population falls into that category. Given the lifetime prevalence of schizophrenia is on average 0.72% (Saha et al., 2005), though with considerable variation through space and time (Saha et al., 2006), when added to the 1% prevalence of psychotic bipolar disorder (Merikangas et al., 2011), the number of 1st and 2nd degree relatives at risk can be calculated from data on the average family size, while taking into account lowered fertility of the proband (Haukka et al., 2003). Some overlap in family member risk might occur between schizophrenia and bipolar 1 pedigrees, but surely not enough to lower the total prevalence of those with a positive family history of psychosis to below 10%. This number represents a lot of individuals to put at risk.

So, even if Johnny *were* predisposed to mental illness, the number of people with first degree (parent) or second degree (grandparent) family history of mental illness would be 10% of the entire U.S. population. That wouldn't be a strong argument for marijuana proponents to hold.

After corresponding with Dr. Miller, I wrote to Sir Robin Murray, a Scottish psychiatrist and Professor of Psychiatric Research at the Institute of Psychiatry, King's College London. I had read many of his studies, and frankly, I didn't expect to get a response because he is ranked as one of the most influential schizophrenia researchers. Murray is part of the Psychosis Research Group at the Institute of Psychiatry, which researches psychotic illnesses. He and his colleagues were among the first to demonstrate that prolonged heavy abuse of marijuana can contribute to the onset of psychosis. Using high-potency marijuana (or what they call "skunk") before the age of 15 particularly increases the risk.

To my delight, Dr. Robin Murray responded to my email in which I'd asked him about the differences between genetic schizophrenia and marijuana onset psychosis. The main points of his response were:

1)   Obviously, one can develop schizophrenia because one has a heavy genetic loading, even if one never smokes cannabis.

2)   One can develop schizophrenia if one smokes lots of cannabis, even if one has no genetic loading for schizophrenia.

3)   It's easiest to develop schizophrenia if one has some genetic vulnerability and also smokes cannabis.

   You might think that it's a bit like heart attacks. You can have a heart attack because you have a heavy genetic/familial loading or because you never take exercise and get very fat in spite of having no genetic loading, but it's easiest if you have genetic loading and get very fat.

Hope this helps.
Robin

So, that's the point. There is no scenario in which cannabis is guaranteed to be harmless for anybody. But we can say that its use increases risk—that is, you could develop schizophrenia even if you never used marijuana. You could use marijuana and develop schizophrenia when you otherwise wouldn't have. You could be genetically inclined to schizophrenia, use marijuana, and develop schizophrenia when you wouldn't have or earlier than you would have. And if you know your child is genetically inclined or already has a mental illness, mood disorder, or genetic predisposition, keep him or her away from marijuana. If your child has none of these things, still keep him or her away from marijuana. Why risk it in any of these scenarios?

I want to emphasize that having certain genes does not automatically cause schizophrenia. Dr. Erik Messamore, a member of Johnny's Ambassadors Scientific Advisory Board, said, "Genetics aren't destiny. You can protect them to avoid mental illness." Genes usually require a trigger— an environmental change that pushes them over the edge. Marijuana can provide that trigger.

Researchers are still in the process of determining which variants react to marijuana use. Dr. Messamore said there are over 100 risk genes that can give rise to schizophrenia, and we all carry a few of them. A recent study[1] suggests carriers with the catechol-O-methyltransferase (COMT) gene variant called valine158 are most likely to develop schizophrenia when exposed to marijuana. COMT is an enzyme responsible for the breakdown of dopamine in the frontal cortex of the brain. Carriers of the COMT valine158 allele (VAL/VAL) were most likely to exhibit psychotic symptoms and develop schizophreniform disorder *if they used cannabis.*

In late 2017, when Johnny was exhibiting behavioral problems from using marijuana, he announced he had developed ADHD and needed to be on medication. So, we took him to a local psychiatric center that administered the Genomind "Genecept Assay® Report" to see if he tested for any problematic genetic conditions. After evaluating him and receiving the results, the counselor told us Johnny definitely did not have ADHD, and Adderall would only serve to make him high. After Johnny died and I learned about the COMT gene as a potential risk factor for schizophrenia, I checked his report. Johnny had the genotype Val/Met, which is normal. He also had a normal C/C gene for the Dopamine 2 receptor, which is affected by dopamine in the brain.

Bottom line, Johnny's grandfather never showed any signs of psychosis, and Johnny never experienced psychosis until years after using marijuana. When Johnny would quit using marijuana, the psychosis would start to go away, but it would return after using it again.

April 20, 2014 — Mom/Dad Agreement

Johnny was highly analytical *and* had excellent verbal skills. We always told him he would be a good lawyer. He was always negotiating "deals" with us — more time playing outside with our dog, Lily, because it was good exercise for her, ten more minutes reading his book before bedtime because it was making him smarter, or five more minutes on his video game until he finished that round because the game would penalize him if he quit early, etc. Very clever guy.

When he turned 14, Johnny wanted expanded privileges as a teenager. To make it official, he suggested we negotiate and sign a "Memorandum of Understanding" between us, outlining the "rules" and "his responsibilities." He claimed this way would prevent any misunderstandings, so we wouldn't have to nag him. You may think this is a bit odd, but we didn't. We were advised by Johnny that a "Behavioral Modification Contract" could be helpful to hold him responsible for his behaviors and accountable to the consequences. This was just how Johnny's brain worked, so we were agreeable to his requests. (No, we didn't create these agreements with our other two children.) Here was the agreement:

Johnny Stack agrees to:

1) Join the STEM program for RCHS and participate in all required activities.

2) Homework must be started at 4:30—no later.

3) Between the time he gets home and 4:30, he will walk Lily for a minimum of 5 minutes and do his chores (weekly on Tuesday, Friday, plus all daily chores as needed), proactively, with no reminders. Additional requests and chores may be given outside his regular chores.

4) ALL homework must be finished for the following day and larger projects before games can be played. Plan homework proactively and don't procrastinate on future due dates.

5) If he has an incomplete, there will be no Wi-Fi privileges and/or gaming until fixed. He may keep his laptop and phone for homework. If Johnny has done everything possible to fix it (late, sick, makeup), games are allowed if an acceptable explanation is given.

6) Research, download, and use an app (or calendar reminders) on the phone for tracking deadlines, schedule, and homework.

7) For the 1st semester of high school, all gaming ends at 10:15, and be in bed by 10:30 (with hygiene items done). This item may be readdressed for second semester, but it's not guaranteed to be changed.

Mom and Dad agree to:

1) Allow Johnny to play on the computer when he gets home from school (assuming someone is here to turn it on) until 4:30, at which time homework begins. Chores must be done, and the dog must be walked prior to 4:30.

2) Purchase an Xbox One and a laptop (perhaps Alienware).

3) Allow Johnny to dis-enroll in archery and track.

4) Allow Johnny to select his bedtime, including eliminating the 8:30 gaming restriction. Allow Johnny to play video games as long as he wants until 10:15, provided all items in this agreement are followed and he's in bed by 10:30.

Both agree to:

1) Never call names or say "you're acting like ..."

2) Hug each other and say, "I love you," at least once a day, even if we are angry.

3) If Johnny doesn't follow through on any item in this agreement, he loses his privileges on all devices (and Wi-Fi turned off) for the rest of the evening. Reminders will not be given, and he will not argue with this punishment.

4) Parents reserve the right to discipline outside of this agreement for additional infractions not listed here. If we tell Johnny we need him, he must respond.

5) This agreement shall be in effect until graduation from high school unless revisions are re-negotiated and mutually agreed. Mom and Dad may revoke this agreement at any time if not consistently followed.

_____

Johnny

_____

Mom

_____

Dad

I still have a copy of the signed version of this agreement hanging with a magnet on a file cabinet in my office. That's where Johnny prominently stuck it so I could easily refer to it.

September 1, 2014 — First High School Party

At 14 years old, Johnny first tried marijuana at a high school party. I know because he came home and told me.

"My friend has a big brother who is 18 years old and has a med card (medical marijuana card). We all wanted to try getting high. I liked it."

As most parents do, we always told our children some variation of the warning, "Don't do drugs of any kind, ever. Drugs will kill your brain cells and make you stupid. If you never try it, you'll never get hooked on it. People only get addicted because they say yes one time, etc., etc., etc." Looking back, knowing what I know now about emotional intelligence, I probably didn't respond with the proper "motivational interviewing" parenting skills. Instead, I got upset at him.

"I TOLD you not to ever try smoking or drugs. We do not allow that in our home."

"Did you ever use marijuana?"

I flashed back to high school. "Yes, which is why it's not allowed in our home because it's going to ruin that beautiful mind of yours and kill your brain cells! Do not do it again."

Many parents think their children start using THC products to combat life's stressors or because they think marijuana isn't as dangerous as other drugs. Maybe they are feeling pressure from their parents to do well in school. Maybe they think it will help them "chill out" and control their stress. Maybe they see their friends use it, and *they* haven't had any problems. Perhaps they're just curious about how it makes them feel, and they are just experimenting. Or like Johnny, perhaps they like getting high, so they get hooked and can't stop.

At this point, I had NO idea about the potency and addiction potential of today's THC products. I didn't understand adolescent brain development. I didn't know use of high-potency marijuana could trigger or cause mental illness. I didn't know today's THC was addicting. My argument was that it would make him stupid. Studies have shown you can lose IQ points with marijuana use, which aligned with my stereotype of the "stoners" when I was in high school versus any real knowledge.

When I laid down the law with Johnny, I thought that would be the end of it because that's how I was raised. In the military culture, I did as I was told. Instead, he just stopped telling me — until he got caught.

September 1, 2015 — Concentrates Arrive at School

Around 2010, hash oil products appeared, and dispensaries began to carry early versions of budders, saps, and waxes. They weren't common when voters voted to legalize recreational marijuana in Colorado in 2012. But by 2015, these new-fangled high-potency waxes and extracts started appearing in high schools. The Colorado Department of Public Health and Environment started tracking "dabbing" on its annual Healthy Kids Colorado Survey (HKCS). I'd never heard of concentrates and didn't know a "dab" of marijuana from a dance move. In fact, it wasn't for another two years until Johnny left for Colorado State University (CSU) that we found a "Nectar Collector" in his dorm room and said, "What is this stuff?"

However, the 2019 HKCS reported 10.2% of high school students are using dabs, and of those who admit to using marijuana, 52% report dabbing—a nearly 70% increase in only two years.

Have you ever heard of dabbing? No, not the hip-hop dance! "Dabs" are extracted concentrates of tetrahydrocannabinol or THC, the chemical (cannabinoid) in marijuana that makes users "high." Here's how dabs are made:

• Cannabis flowers are run through a solvent such as butane, ethanol, or propane.

- The THC leaves the plant material and dissolves into the solvent.
- The concentrated THC solution is filtered to remove (most of) the solvent and dried in a tray.
- The result is a sticky, bronze-colored oily substance that looks like beeswax or earwax.
- These can be additionally processed into distillates, which are more pure THC oils and extracts.
- Dabs are a chemical, not a plant, and they are highly potent, containing up to 99% THC.
- Dabs are typically heated on a hot surface with the vapors inhaled through a dab rig or dab pen.

Dabs are usually called by their consistency, such as shatter, wax, budder, crumble, live resin, or pull 'n snap. Many advocates, usually in states like Colorado and Nevada where recreational marijuana use is legal, defend dabbing as no worse than smoking pot. But they're full of it. Dabbing carries a *lot* more risk for mental illness and addiction than smoking. *And* its levels of THC aren't regulated or restricted.

Dabbing isn't the only way high-potency marijuana is delivered. There's also:

a) **Smoking** — This refers to the dried flowers of the marijuana plant. In practice, it could include seeds, bits of stems, and shredded leaves as well. Users often refer to any cannabis plant matter by the catch-all terms flower, herb, bud, or grass. Until the 1990s, THC potency in herb averaged 3-5%; now, it varies between about 12-25%, depending on the cannabis strain, with an average of 15.6% in 2018.[2] Growers continually increase herb potency through selective breeding, and they boast strains from 30-40% THC. It's usually smoked using a pipe or a bong or rolled into a joint or a blunt.

b) **Eating** (edibles such as candy and brownies) — Edibles are made either directly with the dried flower or with THC concentrates, so potency varies widely. In Colorado, one serving in an edible is measured in milligrams (mg) rather than percentages and is 10 mg per serving, but not all states are regulated. Be aware that one package (such as a candy bar) could contain 1,000 mg or more, so the serving size consumed is extremely important.

c) **Vaping** (such as oil and distillates) — Users vape high-THC oil in a pen. Distillates go through extra refinement processes to remove additional compounds. Once the THC has been distilled, it is re-condensed, and the finished product can be anywhere from 15% to 99% pure THC. Distillates like these are usually vaporized, but users also put them under the tongue, dab them, smoke them, ingest them in a capsule, or infuse them into an edible.

d) **Other products** (such as THC-infused soda, tampons, suppositories, toothpicks, etc.) The pot industry has created countless ways to get THC into the body through any opening.

What you *really* need to know is this — even today's more potent marijuana plants contain 28% THC[3] or higher (with one grower boasting over 40%), while the weed we rolled in the '70s and '80s was 2-5% THC. Dabs, on the other hand, are more than three times more potent than the strongest marijuana plant. *A dab is no longer a plant. Dabs aren't natural; they are CHEMICALS.*

Dab is to marijuana what crack is to cocaine. Depending on potency, one dab is like smoking three to five joints at once. So, for example, an edible brownie contains one serving of THC which is 10 milligrams. If you have a variant like shatter that is 65% THC, one gram is actually 650 milligrams of THC!

The write-up on a bag of "Scooby Snacks Shatter" reads, "There may be long term physical or mental health risks from use of marijuana including additional risks for women who are or may become pregnant or are breastfeeding. Use of marijuana may impair your ability to drive a car or operate machinery. *This product was produced without regulatory oversight for health, safety or efficacy.* This product complies with testing requirements. This packaging is child resistant. This product is intended to be inhaled."

In addition to no regulatory oversight, here's what's worse — dabbing has become popular among young people.[4] Many kids start dabbing by age 14. Most of the time, their parents don't have a clue. You see, dab vapor doesn't have the skunky smell most marijuana smoke has. It may not even have a scent at all, so kids can do it behind their parents' backs at home and their teachers' backs in school. Vaping THC doesn't always make your breath stink in the same way tobacco and grass do, so they don't have to be quite as sneaky. Vaping devices can look just like nicotine vaping devices, so check the cartridges. They may tell you they are "just vaping," but be aware they could be vaping THC. "Vaping" can refer to nicotine or THC while dabbing is only marijuana.

Maybe you think young users are just being typical teens. Maybe you think marijuana is harmless because it's legal. Maybe you think your child is getting straight As, so marijuana can't be affecting him or that it's not your kid because you go to church. Well, I used to think all of that, too.

However, until the mid-to-late 20s, a person's brain is still developing,[5] and intoxicants can damage brain development. Hence, one reason why 21 is the legal age for alcohol, pot, and cigarettes (except "medical marijuana," where the legal age is 18 and an oxymoron) is because people don't actually get a prescription. It's recommended "off label." But numerous medical studies show dabbing can slow mental development and cause depression[6] as well as trigger schizophrenia.[7] And these mental illnesses can lead to suicide.[8]

Johnny only realized that connection weeks before his death.

Compared to heroin or crack, marijuana has a lower addiction rate, but the danger is today's high-potency pot is extremely hazardous to the developing mind. It's highly addictive[9] with dabs being like pot on steroids. There's also a high rate of psychological addiction among young people. Sure, maybe they could stop, but they enjoy the high so much, they don't *want* to stop.

It doesn't take an addiction to dabbing to hurt you. For some who've tried it, it took just *one hit* to put them in the hospital with life-threatening effects or cause psychosis.[10] My 51-year-old girlfriend landed in the mental hospital for three weeks from hallucinations caused from hitting a dab pen twice. This doesn't even account for all the damage dabbers do to their families[11]— often accidentally, sometimes fatally.

In fact, the Retail Marijuana Public Health Advisory Committee (RMPHAC) 2020 report, which is part of the Colorado Department of Public Health and Environment, issued this statement:

> The RMPHAC reviewed the relationships between adolescent and young adult marijuana use and cognitive abilities, academic performance, mental health, and future substance use. Weekly marijuana use by adolescents is associated with deficits in academic and cognitive abilities, even 28 days after last use. Weekly use is also associated with failure to graduate from high school or complete a college degree. Adolescents and young adults who use marijuana are more likely to experience psychotic symptoms as adults

(such as hallucinations, paranoia, and delusional beliefs), future psychotic disorders (such as schizophrenia) and suicidal thoughts or attempting suicide. Evidence shows that adolescents who use marijuana can become addicted to marijuana, and that treatment for marijuana addiction can decrease use and dependence. Additionally, those who quit using marijuana have lower risks of adverse cognitive and mental health outcomes than those who continue to use. Marijuana use is also associated with future use and use disorder for tobacco, alcohol, and other drugs. Adolescent use of marijuana with higher THC concentration (>10% THC) is associated with continued use and development of future mental health symptoms and disorders.

A joint study from the University of Michigan and Brown University[12] found higher potency marijuana to be more addictive than lower potencies. It is associated with a higher risk of cannabis use disorder (CUD) or marijuana addiction in young users. Researchers found that regular pot users who first tried marijuana when the national average THC levels held at 4.9% had almost twice the increased risk of developing symptoms of cannabis use disorder within a year. But those who started regularly using pot when national average THC levels were 12.3% had a 4.8 times higher risk of cannabis use disorder. And yet the state of Colorado continues to allow these high-potency THC products to be sold with no regulation or limitation on potency.

In a nutshell, marijuana harms adolescents in these ways:
1) Marijuana dependence[13]

2) Decreased IQ[14]

3) Increased risk of addiction with higher potency[15]

4) Increased odds of using other drugs[16]

5) Death from throwing up[17]

6) More likely to drop out of school[18]

7) Possible psychosis and schizophrenia[19]

8) Decreased fertility rates[20]

9) Lowered motivation to do things[21]

10) Possible paranoia and thoughts that others intend to harm you[22]

11) Health damages[23]

12) Poor driving skills[24]

September 1, 2016 — Junior Year

Fast forward two years to Johnny's junior year of high school. He was driving, so it was harder for us to track his comings and goings. In the fall, Johnny had his first "real" girlfriend and seemed to genuinely care about her. His girlfriend said, "It was just like any other high school relationship and ended just like most. Frankly, he wasn't very nice to me at the end, so I don't recall all the memories since unfortunately we left on a bad note." In a seven-month period, he went from a nice, sweet kid who would sit on the couch and snuggle with her while watching movies and dressing up as nerds for Halloween to being a jerk to his girlfriend. He took her to prom because he'd committed and then broke up with her right afterward. He hid his use from her and treated her badly. In fact, his marijuana use made him treat many friends poorly. Several of them came up to me at the funeral, apologetically saying, "Johnny and I weren't on speaking terms at the end, but . . ."

He continued to get As in school but started procrastinating more and didn't seem motivated to learn like he used to be. He played a lot of a video game called Counter-Strike: Global Offensive (CS:GO) with his buddies and achieved the highest rank. Knowing he was interested in becoming a game designer, computer programmer, or computer engineer, I didn't say much about the hours he'd spend playing video games. The summer before his junior year in high school, we enrolled him in Stanford University for a two-week "Level Design with Counterstrike: Global Offensive Academy" program which he really enjoyed.

While this was happening, Johnny continued to hide his marijuana use from us. We found out later from Snapchat photos that the little cartridges he told us contained nicotine actually contained THC oil. He was refilling them and smoking marijuana right under our noses, but we were clueless. I feel sad about how ignorant I was. It never occurred to me to test the little bottles of juice and cartridges he said were "just nicotine."

One morning, I went into his room before school and saw a telltale haze in the air.

"Johnny, what in the world is this? It's like a jungle in here! You know there is no vaping allowed in the house!"

"Mom, it's no big deal. Everyone does it."

"I don't care what everyone else does. You know the rules of the household. We will withdraw driving and phone privileges if you do it again."

I told John what happened, and while Johnny was at school, we searched his room. Sure enough, we found a green glass pipe and a small butane torch, like one you'd use for crème brûlée. Why

I didn't think the torch was odd, I don't know. We confronted him when he came home from school.

"Johnny, do you have an explanation for these items?"

"Those aren't mine, Mom. They are my friend's."

"Oh, really? I don't believe you for one minute. Maybe we should call your friend and his mom together and talk about it."

"Mom, please don't do that to me. You're going to make him hate me if you throw me under the bus like that."

"Johnny, we have a very firm rule in this household—no marijuana! Come with us."

John took the pipe out to the cement patio and smashed it. Then we grounded him and took away his car for a time. We didn't know what else to do.

His disobedience got much worse. John bought a car tracker and started keeping tabs on his whereabouts. His stories of what he was doing, who he was with, and where he was going didn't add up. For example, we'd ask him to pick up James from baseball practice, but we could see he was at his girlfriend's house instead of the baseball field. Or he would be at an unknown location when he was supposed to be at a friend's house. We confronted him, but he'd just lie. We took away his car, so he refused to go to school, and slowly, his grades started to slip. He thought we were tracking his phone, and he didn't know about the car tracker for a long time. Then he suddenly found out about it (we didn't know how) and smashed the device in the driveway. (He later admitted to us that he had installed a keylogger on John's computer. No wonder he always knew the password to the Wi-Fi router, so he and James could get up after we went to bed and play video games.)

On December 12, 2016, he wrecked my 2001 Honda Odyssey minivan. It was old but reliable, and he had learned to drive on it. We let him drive it to school and to pick up his brother. One night, he was driving James home from baseball practice. He drove into a construction zone, and the cones suddenly narrowed from two lanes to one. He was going too fast and hit the car in front of him. Everyone was fine physically, but the cars were totaled. Since Johnny rear-ended the other driver, our insurance rates increased. I didn't know until later that Johnny routinely drove while high. His therapist, whose name was also John, told me Johnny had driven to his office for an appointment and was so high that he got lost and couldn't find the office he'd been to many times. He was so high that his therapist made him sit there for three hours before he could leave, or he would call the police.

After Johnny passed, I discovered several videos he took of himself driving and smoking marijuana. It's likely he hit the other car that night because he was high. He had James in the car with him, and he could have killed them both as well as the occupants of the other car.

From the "THC Concentration in Colorado Marijuana Health Effects and Public Health Concerns" report dated July 30, 2020, high-school-aged youth are twice as likely to drive after using marijuana than after using alcohol. The report also found a significant 24% increase in high schoolers admitting to driving after consuming marijuana in the past month.

Knowing what I know now, I look back and can see these obvious signs. You might be shaking your head at me right now, wondering how I missed all of this. I simply thought he was being a moody, sullen, not-so-nice, hormonal teenager. Not having experience with marijuana, I didn't know he was having a problem with it.

After he died, several of his friends came over to us. One admitted he was the "leader of the pack" who most likely got Johnny involved in marijuana. He asked for our forgiveness. I flashed back to Johnny telling me about him being sent to long-term rehab for psychosis. Thankfully, he recovered and was better now. He admitted to us he still struggled to stay sober.

If your child becomes a regular user, you might think it would be obvious, but that's not necessarily so. It can be easy for your teen to hide it from you, but you *do* have behavioral cues. For one, Johnny's personality started to change. He became moody and lacked motivation. He no longer wanted to participate in any extracurricular activities and kept withdrawing to his bedroom to be alone. I would question him about the amount of time spent playing video games and ask him to come down to enjoy time with the family. His attitude was basically, "Mom, I'm getting straight As, so leave me alone. This is what I want to do for a living." He became increasingly irritable, and his friends started referring to him as "salty." He stopped doing his chores and no longer followed household rules. He would stand defiantly in the hallway, vape, and blow it into the air. At times, he would complain of random stomach aches and the need to stay home from school. Then he would sit at the kitchen table at breakfast and kind of groan and hold his head. When I asked what was wrong, he'd say, "I just have a headache."

Like all substance use disorders, cannabis use disorder (CUD) comes with a suite of telltale withdrawal symptoms. Cannabis withdrawal syndrome (CWS) is a clinical indicator of CUD, and it's one of the factors that's convinced most health care professionals that marijuana is, in fact, addictive. Generations of users and proponents have insisted the opposite. Perhaps it wasn't addictive with "old-fashioned" marijuana, but this argument no longer applies for today's modern herb with its 15-40% THC content and extracts with 90%+ THC content.

Admittedly, CWS does tend to be mild compared to withdrawal syndromes for meth, cocaine, heroin, and other commonly abused drugs—though the sufferer won't perceive it's mild while suffering through withdrawal. However, as long as the user completely abstains, the negative effects start to reverse within two days, and CWS can subside within a month.[25] If they tough out the worst effects, users can walk away from marijuana for good, if they choose. However, some irreparable damage with long-term repercussions may remain, as we'll discuss.

Unfortunately, when CWS starts to manifest, users may treat it with marijuana.[26] After all, it *does* make them feel better which is what happens in addiction. This can result in a repetitive, vicious cycle. If you're concerned your child is abusing marijuana, this is why you should know the withdrawal symptoms.

Anyone who's ever lived with teenagers knows how moody they can be. Unfortunately, some of those moods are similar to certain symptoms of CWS, so take care when "diagnosing" your child. Don't focus on behavioral or mood issues alone. Realize that cannabis withdrawal symptoms can include:

- Poor and decreased appetite

- Mood changes

- Irritability

- Insomnia and other sleep difficulties

+ Headaches

+ Inability to concentrate

+ Excessive sweating, including cold sweats

+ Chills

+ Increased depression

+ Stomach problems

+ Nausea

+ Vomiting

One set of researchers from Queens University in Ontario conducted a meta-analysis of 47 studies including 23,518 individuals.[27] The researchers concluded that the prevalence of CWS for those patients after abstinence was 47%, indicating *almost half* of all former regular and dependent users fulfilled a definitive indicator for CUD.

A similar meta-analysis of 21 studies[28] was published in *Addictive Behaviors* in October 2020. It revealed a 22% chance of users developed CUD on average (rising to 33% for those who started using in adolescence), while 13% presented with cannabis dependence, and 13% suffered from cannabis addiction.

Not all observers have been persuaded by the earlier study, however. Proponents of marijuana argued that the sample universe was improperly selected, and many of the studies were conducted so differently that the ultimate results could not be generalized to all marijuana users.[29] The author of this Harvard Medical School blog has a point; however, unless I'm missing some methodological nuance, it seems remarkable that two separate peer-reviewed meta-studies in 2020 (one of which had not been published at the time of his commentary) produced such similar results.

CWS—and cannabis withdrawal symptoms in general—may prove hard to see through the teenage "fog of war" caused by normal parents-aren't-cool, hormone- and peer-driven behavior. All kids have their bad moods and tummy aches. But the possibility they might result from CUD, a serious disorder, makes them worth looking at closely.

In a young person, CUD is an indicator of a lifestyle choice causing lifelong disabilities that can not only hurt your teen but can tear your family apart. It can even take your child by suicide (like Johnny) or result in life-long mental illness. Unfortunately, cannabis withdrawal symptoms aren't necessarily a one-time thing, and neither is CUD. They can come and go, depending on availability of supply, the user's ability to afford marijuana, and most poignantly, *when* users decide to fight their addiction to weed.

Teens can prove to be smart about hiding their drug use. The only way parents might learn about it is through a slip-up, such as finding it in their room or seeing withdrawal symptoms. If you observe more than a few of the symptoms in the list that you can't otherwise explain or if they seem to occur repeatedly or suddenly, ask your child directly, "Are you using marijuana or dabbing?" Then watch the reaction. If he or she refuses to go to the doctor or do an in-home THC test, this should arouse your suspicion. Remember, until teens reach the age of 18, you have a right to have your children tested for drugs when you take them in for a medical exam. If you're 100% wrong and they are clean, it's better to risk them being annoyed at you than suffer a permanent long-term disability. You can always apologize and take them on a shopping trip or to Chick-fil-A for good behavior!

So how do you know if your child is acting like a normal teenager or you're seeing cannabis use? Here are ten true-or-false statements covering the most likely tip-offs that your teen is using marijuana, followed by the answers.

True or False?

1) If my teen used marijuana, I'd be able to smell it.

2) My teen often has red, bloodshot eyes and uses eye drops frequently which could indicate marijuana use.

3) My teen has suddenly changed his circle of friends, but this can't signal possible marijuana use.

4) If my teen is vomiting a lot, it can be a sign of marijuana use.

5) My teen is more lethargic and sleeping more than usual which could signal marijuana use.

6) I found hollowed-out cigars and burned nails in my son's backpack, which seems odd, but they can't be related to marijuana use.

7) If my teen's grades have started to plunge, marijuana could be the cause.

8) My teen seems to be anxious and depressed, but that's just normal teen behavior, not a sign of marijuana use.

9) My teen is saying some strange things about her phone being bugged; this sudden paranoia can indicate marijuana use.

10) I'm not worried about my daughter because teen girls rarely use marijuana.

Answers

1) FALSE — While smoked marijuana has a distinctive, skunky smell, vaped marijuana,[30] whether in oil or solid form, often has little or no smell. You won't be able to smell it on your teen's breath and clothes, and the vapors can easily dissipate in a well-ventilated place. Teens can use a "sploof," which is a handmade filter made from a cardboard tube and a dryer

sheet. A room deodorizer or incense can also effectively mask the smell of marijuana, and your teen may wear more perfume or cologne than normal.

2) TRUE — Marijuana users often have very bloodshot eyes because marijuana is a vasodilator.[31] It lowers your blood pressure which causes the capillaries in your eyes to relax and increases the blood flow to those vessels. To counter this effect, users often use eye drops specially formulated for redness which decreases the size of the capillaries in the eyes to make the bloodshot appearance go away. If you note your teen using a lot of eye drops for no apparent reason or you find bottles of eye drops and don't know why, he or she may be using marijuana.

3) FALSE — Your teen suddenly changing a circle of friends may signal marijuana use. If his friends all use drugs or old friends who don't do drugs no longer associate with your teen, that's another red flag.

4) TRUE — Marijuana toxicity[32] is unexplained nausea and vomiting, increased blood pressure, fast heartbeat, anxiety, panic, paranoia, hallucinations, delusions, and extreme confusion. If your child is vomiting frequently and taking a lot of hot showers, it may be a sign of cannabis hyperemesis syndrome[33] and requires medical treatment. A teen user may also act giddy or "out of it" for no obvious reason or let personal hygiene go.

5) TRUE — Marijuana is known to make users more lethargic. This may manifest as them no longer taking an interest in activities they once enjoyed. An abrupt change in behavior is a classic sign of drug use. If your child suddenly becomes overly tired,[34] combative, secretive, uncommunicative, or loses interest in once-favorite activities, then investigate further.

6) FALSE — Having paraphernalia[35] around the house (and possibly blaming a friend) is a sign of marijuana use. Those hollowed-out cigars you found in your kid's backpacks are used for smoking pot. Users call them blunts.[36] They pack them with herb marijuana and smoke them like regular cigars. They contain a lot more marijuana than a joint and can be very potent. If your child has been hiding burned nails, they're probably dabbing.[37] This highly dangerous form of marijuana use involves inhaling the smoke from burned high-THC concentrates like shatter, budder, and wax. Using nails to hold the marijuana and a lighter to burn it is a simple form of dabbing, though there are "rigs" and pens made specifically for dabbing.

7) TRUE — Teen marijuana users often lose interest in school[38] and may start to skip classes or whole days. It can take a lot of time to be involved in marijuana. They may also stop studying which is reflected in poor grades. Long term, it can lead to a permanent drop in IQ. Like my son Johnny, some users can still function well enough to get by. There are other factors that can cause a drop in academic performance, from emotional distress to physical and psychological problems, but definitely question marijuana use as well.

8) FALSE — Your teen may tell you he or she is using marijuana to "chill out" or as "medicine" for anxiety and depression. However, there's solid scientific evidence that marijuana can cause or worsen these conditions. Marijuana use can definitely trigger depression,[39] and regular users have twice the normal risk[40] for developing it. It can also trigger anxiety[41] or heighten existing anxiety. Meanwhile, anxiety may increase between uses,[42] and anxiety attacks may occur while using.[43]

9) TRUE — Among other things, marijuana can cause psychosis,[44] paranoia,[45] schizophrenia,[46] and suicidal tendencies and thoughts.[47] If you notice any such behavior, investigate it further (or get immediate medical attention if suicidal intent is expressed) because it may be caused by marijuana use.

10) FALSE — Although it's true that fewer females use marijuana than males, marijuana does not respect gender. Some argue females aren't as comfortable with marijuana use as males or males are just more adventurous or more likely to do dangerous things. The truth is that according to the 2014[48] and 2018[49] National Surveys of Drug Use, those who had used in the last month and last year were, on average, 39-43% female. That's not much of a minority; girls use marijuana *almost* as often as boys.

If 20,000+ articles and reports about the negative effects of marijuana aren't enough to convince skeptics of marijuana's harmful nature, perhaps the field guide of the psychiatric profession will. The *Diagnostic and Statistical Manual of Mental Disorders, Fifth Edition* (commonly known as DSM-5), published by the American Psychiatric Association, recognizes CUD/MUD as a genuine SUD. In the opinion of mental health professionals—the people who spend their lives studying and treating ailments of the human mind—marijuana is, in fact, addictive. Some say it's just as addictive[50] as some of the most powerful narcotics as well as its closest competitors, alcohol and tobacco.

The definitive answer lies in the 11 diagnostic indicators of cannabis use (marijuana use) disorders, according to DSM-5.[51] The indicators include:

1) Taking the substance in larger amounts or for longer than intended.

2) Wanting to cut down or stop using the substance but not managing to.

3) Spending a lot of time getting, using, or recovering from use of the substance.

4) Cravings and urges to use the substance.

5) Not managing to do what you should at work, home, or school because of substance use.

6) Continuing to use, even when it causes problems in relationships.

7) Giving up important social, occupational, or recreational activities because of substance use.

8) Using substances again and again, even when it puts you in danger.

9) Continuing to use, even when you know you have a physical or psychological problem that could have been caused or made worse by the substance.

10) Needing more of the substance to get the effect you want (tolerance).

11) Development of withdrawal symptoms which can be relieved by taking more of the substance.

I don't have space to review all 11 diagnostic criteria here, but some marijuana users do exhibit some, many, or even all these criteria. A user doesn't have to experience all 11 of the criteria to have an SUD. At some point though, I saw ALL of them in action during Johnny's struggle with marijuana.

The DSM-5 classifies SUD indicators into four categories:

Criteria	Category
1-4	Impaired Control
5-7	Social Impairment
8-9	Risky Use
10-11	Pharmacological Indicators of Tolerance and Withdrawal

The criteria don't have to show up in order, and some SUD sufferers may not have some of the symptoms.

The DSM-5 also provides guidelines regarding the levels of severity for an SUD:

Number of Symptoms	Level of Severity
2-3	Mild
4-5	Moderate
6+	Severe (dependence/addiction)

So, yes, *marijuana is addictive.* It wouldn't have a medically defined SUD if it weren't. In fact, it's as easily categorized as the opioid SUD or the alcohol SUD, and it acts on the same reward pathway. It can also prove deadly, as I know all too well.

From non-profits to hospitals to private programs, Ben Cort has been a leader inside many forms of addiction treatment and prevention. From 2017 to 2020, Ben was a consultant to various treatment programs, state governments, professional and collegiate athletics, and labor. Today, he is the CEO of Foundry Steamboat Springs, an inpatient treatment program for men in the mountains of Colorado. His TED talk, "Surprising Truths about Legalizing Cannabis," has been viewed over 2.5 million times.

Ben Cort told Johnny's Ambassadors:

The old 80-20 rule has always taught us that for addictive substances in this country, such as alcohol and tobacco, about 80% of the product is purchased by about 20% of the consumers. So, the analogy I like to give is my wife and her couple of margaritas a year mean nothing to the alcohol industry. However, the guy who founded Mad Dog 2020 when he was 12 years old was a solid prospect for the future.

In Colorado, we actually have decent data about this. From the 2019 Colorado Marijuana Enforcement Division annual report, we saw that about 6.1% of all of marijuana users in Colorado purchase 75% of the THC products in the state. I would say that every single one of them would meet the diagnostic criteria for severe substance use disorder. If a small percentage is purchasing three quarters of all of the product in this state, we'd all better recognize that the industry knows that better than we do. They know who their customers are and who's actually paying the bills. That 6.1% better be cultivated so that they can keep them engaged, and they had better be drawn into purchasing more. They've got to do everything they can to add numbers to that and get users hooked at a younger age.

As we can very plainly see by that statistic, the profit of the marijuana industry is driven by addiction and addiction potential. Big marijuana is no different from big tobacco, big alcohol, and big drugs from south of the border.

A 2020 study in the *Journal of Addictive Behaviors*[52] indicates that people who use cannabis have a one in five risk of developing a CUD. Risks increase if cannabis is initiated early and used frequently. Let's assume Johnny used on the "low" end, perhaps once or twice a week on weekends with his buddies. That means he used 50 to 100 times a year!

The risk of developing CUD increases to 33% among young people who have engaged in regular (weekly or daily) use of cannabis. That means one in three youth who start using marijuana while they're young will experience one of these six disorders:

1) Affective disorders of thought and feeling, including bipolar disorder, anxiety disorders, and depression

2) Schizophrenia

3) Amotivational syndrome

4) Disruptive cognitive function

5) Neuropsychological decline

6) Psychotic disorders

In September 2020, the Substance Abuse and Mental Health Services Administration (SAMHSA) released its 2019 Annual National Survey on Drug Use and Health[53] (NSDUH), the most comprehensive drug use survey in the U.S. It told us that out of children ages 12 to 17, 17.2% say they used marijuana in the past year. (In legalized states including Colorado, the percentage is even higher.) Among young adults ages 18 to 25, past-year marijuana users increased from 29.8% (or 9.2 million people) in 2002 to 35.4% (or 12 million people) in 2019. Sadly, in 2019, approximately 699,000 youth ages 12 to 17 had a known addiction to marijuana. They represent 187,000 youth with a new cannabis use disorder (CUD) in 2019 versus 2018. That means more than 500 youth a day have been developing a new CUD in the U.S.!

We've learned that the earlier one starts using marijuana, the higher the risk for addiction. Cannabis use disorder (CUD) shows a general upward trend of use from ages 12 to 18 years. Then at age 19, the rate drops considerably to 8% and steadily declines across the young adult age groups. Given the data, I fear that the changing—and inaccurate—views about marijuana's relative harmlessness may tempt teens to give in to peer pressure and try it at younger and younger ages.

After Johnny died, our friend John Sileo (how many guys named "John" do I have in my life?), an expert in cybercrime, helped us get into Johnny's phone by guessing the password. Johnny had written down two pages of accounts, logins, and passwords in his journal, but he didn't write down the phone password, perhaps intentionally. So, we sent photos of the pages to John Sileo, who figured out the password. We are eternally grateful to him as we were locked out and couldn't do it ourselves. We found a tab in the Snapchat app called "for your eyes only," and thankfully, the same password worked there. We were shocked to discover years of photos and videos showing Johnny and his friends using marijuana.

February 7, 2017 — Updated Contract

In the second semester of his junior year, it became clear another Behavioral Modification Contract was in order once Johnny turned 17. This time it *wasn't* his idea. We only had one year left until he turned 18. I wish we would have known about drug testing then because we would have required drug testing as a condition of this agreement to ensure he was adhering to the third item.

Johnny will:

- Follow the rules of the house until he leaves home for college, understanding that privileges (such as driving, technology, and phone usage) may be withdrawn if broken.

- Adhere to curfew (increase to 10:00 on school nights and 12:00 on weekends).

- Not drink or use marijuana.

- Not vape nicotine in the house.

- Go to (girlfriend's) house only when a parent is present; follow the rule that a parent must be present at all friends' parties.

- Notify parents of your location.

- Update our shared Google calendar with tutoring hours and personal plans.

- Pay $133/month for insurance (currently—may go up after court date in February if USAA raises it). Due on the 1st of the month in cash or transfer from checking or savings.

- Pay for his own gas, recreation, and purchases (with personal debit card).

- Take care of the dog: daily walk, poop duty, and fill food and water bowls.

- Complete "extra" requests without complaint (such as taking down Christmas lights, bringing in groceries, or taking Grandma to the store, if requested).

- Attend family activities and special occasions as requested.

Mom and Dad will:
- Provide a roof over your head and food.

- Provide car maintenance.

- Provide health and car insurance.

- Provide phone service, television, and internet access.

- Provide additional items as requested and deemed necessary.

- Give Johnny $5/day per school day for food.

- No longer provide an allowance.

- Arrange to have Johnny's previous chores completed.

- Arrange to have James driven to activities OR pay Johnny $5 upon request (if he's available).

- Pay for college tuition, room, and board at an in-state university for four years upon successful graduation from high school.

August 11, 2017 —
First Semester of Senior Year

Johnny hated it when I bragged about him, but I can brag about him now that he's gone. The summer before his senior year of high school, he took the SAT exam and got a perfect score on the math portion (800/800) and a 1430 overall. Then he took the ACT and scored a 34 (a perfect score is a 36), to which he complained about the poor wording on some of the answers in the English section. (Looking back, I wonder how he would have scored if he *weren't* using marijuana.)

As a parent, it was easy to rationalize, "Well, he did so well on these assessments, so he can't be having problems." Or "He's getting straight As, has a 4.0 GPA, and got a scholarship, so maybe the marijuana isn't affecting him much." By the end of his senior year, after nearly failing the last semester with four Ds, his GPA was still so high that he graduated with honors. Don't let good grades fool you!

When Johnny's senior year started, a sign of worse things to come came on August 23, 2017, when the home phone rang at 3:30 a.m. I woke up in a fog and heard the last ring as it went to voicemail. I told myself it was probably a telemarketer but decided I'd better check. Sure enough, I heard this message, "Hi, Mr. Stack. This is Debbie Graber with Douglas County Sheriff's office. I am out with your son at the dog park off South Havana, and it is 3:30 in the morning. So, if you could call me back, we can kind of figure where we can go from here. I will try back shortly." John went to get our son. Johnny's story was he had left in the middle of the night to comfort a friend who was having personal problems. We took his car for two weeks. He hated riding the bus.

Since he was now getting into legal trouble, we engaged a therapist, John Davis of 2Xtreme (another John, yes). He met with Johnny and then met with us separately and confirmed Johnny was "breaking all the rules."

On September 23, 2017, his high school held its homecoming. Instead of coming home by midnight, Johnny didn't come home that night at all. I assume he couldn't because he was high and/or drunk. He breezily walked in the following morning as if nothing had happened. This time, we took the car away for three days which we thought was a light consequence. We told him he broke curfew and didn't call us, and we were worried. He said that he was a senior and shouldn't have to be home by midnight.

Johnny became exceedingly angry over the three-day loss of his car. We thought that was an overreaction as he'd earned that penalty. He argued with us about it the following day, and when we refused to give the car back, he went up to his room, packed his suitcase, and left. We didn't know where he went. We guessed he'd likely be able to couch surf with friends for a little while. One mom reached out to me about letting him stay there. That lasted one night as he got into a huge fight with a good friend. We got concerned when we didn't hear from him for several days. The phone tracker app showed him up in north Denver at an unknown location (now we assume a marijuana dealer). So, with the help of his therapist, we wrote Johnny a letter.

CHAPTER 3:

THE DESCENT

September 27, 2017 — Ultimatum

Johnny,

I hope that you've had some time to think since you chose to pack your suitcase and leave on Monday night. I know your father and I have. We are disappointed with the way you chose to separate but can't keep you from leaving. We love you and pray you choose to live at home again, but we can't make you.

If you do not choose to live at home again, you need to understand this is not a hotel, and you can't come and go as you please. You need to either live at home or live elsewhere, permanently. There is no open-door policy; you may not walk into our home if you forget or want something. You must get permission to come inside.

So, we are setting a boundary that if you choose not to come home by MONDAY, OCTOBER 2 at 8:00 p.m., you are choosing to move out of the house without our support. We will be changing the locks on the doors, garage pads, and remote controls, and if you enter our home, we will report you to the police for breaking and entering. We will pack up the items in your bedroom and leave them on the front porch, and you may come pick them up. We are currently providing your car insurance, which we will no longer provide. We are currently providing your phone service, which we will no longer provide. We will no longer be providing you with money for gas, food, clothes, or any expenses. We will continue to provide your health insurance and support your schooling. We will pay for college only if you graduate in May 2018.

If you do choose to live at home again, we will continue to provide you with a bedroom, food, clothing, car insurance, phone service, and gas money. Your privileges will be suspended until such a time as you can prove you're not using. You must agree to be drug tested at will to verify you're following this house rule. You will lose an additional week plus three days of driving privileges for staying out all night on homecoming. You will continue to follow the midnight curfew on weekends and 10:00 p.m. on weekdays. While you live at home, you must keep us informed of your whereabouts, including the name of whom you're with and if you're spending the night, the address of your location. You will continue to perform your chores and family responsibilities.

We will wait to hear your decision.

Love,
Mom and Dad

At 8:02 p.m., Johnny calmly walked in the door. "I will agree to follow the rules," he stated flatly. We didn't follow through on the drug testing, however, and that's a big regret of mine. Our primary care doctor was resistant to giving him a drug test because Johnny refused when they asked for his consent. We were unaware you could do tests at home with kits, and the doctor didn't offer that information. There's so much I know now that I wish I knew then.

We missed the opportunity to send him to a residential treatment program. Looking back, before he turned 18 was the time for an intervention. Of course, I didn't know he would die, but not sending him away before it was too late is something I regret now. In hindsight, there are all kinds of things we wish we'd done but couldn't have known. We did the best we could at the time and made the best decisions we could with the information we had.

January 16, 2018 — Second Semester of Senior Year

Johnny continued to be defiant and started missing school. At the beginning of the second semester, he basically told his counselor he would be 18 on February 7, so I couldn't require him to attend school as he'd be an adult. He advised the school to discontinue our access to his school portal, so we couldn't see his grades or how much school he was missing.

A few weeks before his birthday, we received the following letter from the school, outlining an "Attendance Plan":

The purpose of this plan is to clarify certain duties (commitments) of the student, the parent, and the school regarding school attendance. It is also to assess both family and student concerns and needs that when addressed will result in better school attendance. This Plan will continue to be developed from time to time and, if attendance does not improve and legal action is taken by the school district, serve to inform the Court on the status of the student, the interventions attempted, and results attained.

87 School Days to Date
21 Unexcused Absences
35 Total Absences

At this point, I just wanted Johnny to finish high school. I remember thinking, "We just need to get through high school. He'll graduate, go to college on his scholarship, and meet some new people, and he will be okay." I really had my head in the sand and practiced a lot of wishful thinking.

As a last-ditch effort to get him to attend school regularly and do his homework, we confiscated his laptop. We told him he was to use the desktop in my office for his homework, and he wasn't allowed to play his video games until his grades and attendance had improved. He got so angry that he got physical. He entered my bedroom, demanded his laptop back, and shoved me. John was in the master bathroom. As he turned the corner, he saw the entire action. John has a second-degree black belt in karate, so Johnny found himself flat on his back in about two seconds. John yelled at him and told him he was to never put his hands on me again. This was clearly a volatile situation and an unhealthy environment for our younger son James, who was still at home and witnessing these interactions.

The following morning when Johnny was in the shower, we searched his backpack and found a glass pipe and a little bag of ten Adderall pills. We confronted him about these items. He admitted he bought the pills for $1 each from a classmate "to help him study." I threw the pills in the toilet, broke the pipe, and threw it away. Johnny swore at me, "F*** you, f***ing c***." Hearing that, I had a bit of a meltdown and started sobbing. John told him to leave. It was *hell* all the time.

John and I decided that due to his continued marijuana use, his defiance, the pushing incident, his refusal to go to school or accept correction, and now his verbal and emotional abuse, he needed to move out of the house when he turned 18. He was simply not safe to have in the home, and we still had James to think about.

When Johnny returned home, we had a very calm conversation with him. We told him that when he turned 18, we wanted to reach a mutual decision that it was best for him to leave our home due to his continued marijuana use and refusal to follow the family rules. He was surprised but did not disagree. We told him we loved him and wanted to help him get help when he was ready. The money he had saved for the past 18 years (nearly $5,000) that was earmarked as spending money for his four years of college, we would transfer to his checking account. He could use it for rent and expenses until he left for college. We would pay for his phone and car insurance if he agreed to see his therapist weekly, and everything else was on his own. If he graduated from high school, we would still pay the college expenses not covered by the scholarship. He agreed. I was sad to my core that we'd arrived at this place, but we simply couldn't allow him to stay at home and use marijuana.

March 1, 2018 — Moves Out

With a heavy heart, we helped Johnny look for a room to rent that was close to us and his school. I wish we had known about sober living facilities or an Oxford House.[54] We would have encouraged him to move into one of those, but we settled on a home with a room for rent a couple miles down the road from us.

The landlord was an air marshal, so we thought, "Great, he's in law enforcement! If Johnny gets out of line, he'll call the cops on him." Nope.

Once, his landlord actually said to me on the phone, "I think Johnny is selling weed or drugs from the house. There is a constant stream of people going from their cars to his bedroom window."

I said, "What!? Geez, call the police!" He didn't. I guess he needed the rent, and he didn't want to get Johnny in trouble.

At the time, we didn't have access to Johnny's phone, so we couldn't see the selfie he took of himself a couple weeks later dated March 15, 2018, driving to get his med card. The caption said (spelling and grammatical error included), "Anyone wanna smoke me up before I my med card?"

I recently had a long conversation with a friend of his who went to IdRaHaJe Christian Camp with him. Coincidentally, they were later on the same hall and floor at the University of Northern Colorado. She confirmed Johnny had a med card and bought his high-THC distillates from a dispensary. She said he hit a small dab pen frequently throughout the day like it was vape. He had another small water pipe he used for concentrates.

Once we had access to his phone, we were able to login to all of his other devices, computers, and apps, and we found quite a bit of shocking information. One of the photos was of him driving three other young adolescents who looked to be 13 or 14—the same age Johnny was when he started using marijuana. Johnny had come full circle. He became the local school marijuana dealer. That broke my heart. I felt so bad for those boys and their parents, none of whom I knew. I prayed that none of them suffered the same outcome as Johnny.

Most of the photos were selfies using marijuana and his "friends" using marijuana. There were also photos of other drugs in little baggies and stacks of money, confirming he also started dealing during that time. Teens with med cards often become involved in dealing (like my son's first dealer) because they can access marijuana when those under 21 can't, so they sell to them.

I didn't know what all the drugs in the pictures were, so I sent them to my friend and fellow National Marijuana Initiative Speakers Bureau member, Ben Cort. He told me, "The orange pill is a benzo called Alprazolam. The white pill is Oxy, not sure of the mg amount. The capsule is a stimulant called Amphetamine/dextroamphetamine. The gelatin on the foil is LSD. The diversity of those drugs and the quantity suggest that he was dealing. The most telling pic is the one with the coupon and all the weed products. There's no way that was personal use; he had to be reselling after buying with the med card using coupons. Everything else is just a different form of concentrated THC."

So, does a regulated pot industry keep marijuana away from our 18-year-old kids? NO, NO, and NO. The opposite is true. It allows them to deal drugs to younger kids, no black market needed. Teens can't get tobacco or alcohol legally, but they *can* obtain a medical marijuana card without parental knowledge or approval. Then they just need to find a "pot shop" doctor who will sell the minds and souls of children for a few hundred dollars. All they care about is money, not the health and mental well-being of our kids.

Dr. Libby Stuyt is an addiction psychiatrist at the Pueblo Community Health Center, a clinical faculty member of the CU School of Medicine Department of Psychiatry, and one of Johnny's Ambassadors Scientific Advisory Board members.

Dr. Stuyt wrote an op-ed in *MedPage Today* called "Children and 'Medical' Marijuana." I've included several facts summarized here:

* An 18-year-old adolescent in Colorado (whose brain is not yet fully developed and cannot purchase tobacco or alcohol legally) can obtain a medical marijuana card without parental knowledge or approval.
* The physician is not required to write a "prescription," just a recommendation.
* The physician doesn't specify and monitor the type of product, route of administration, amount used, frequency of use, and period of use.
* There is no requirement for follow-up appointments to determine whether the recommendation has been helpful or if there are side effects, only an annual renewal.
* Teens can then take the card to the dispensary and get anything they want or is recommended by the person selling the products—budtenders—who have no requirements for medical training.
* Patients can purchase twice as much in the medical dispensary (2 ounces per day) versus recreational dispensary (1 ounce per day), and it is less expensive because of lower taxes.

◆ Regardless, as of February 2021 in Colorado, there is no tracking ability or any way to see if someone is going from dispensary to dispensary and purchasing more product, a process known as "looping."

◆ The doctor is protected, so you can't find out who gave med cards to them. (If I could only find the creep who gave my perfectly healthy child a med card, I would confront and sue him/her. But their identities are concealed and not even printed on the card.)

Dr. Stuyt's article continued: "The initial rules and regulations required that the recommending doctor have a bona fide physician-patient relationship and that the patient have a debilitating medical condition. However, in the fall of 2009, it was recognized, that although 900 doctors had written approval letters (7% of licensed MDs), just 15 doctors had written 72% of the forms, and FIVE had written fully half. One doctor signed 3,500 letters in a two-day period. This resulted in new legislation further defining a bona fide relationship and limiting physicians authorized to approve cards to those with unrestricted medical and DEA licenses."

Do you think that helped? Nope. Go to many concerts in Colorado, and you'll see a trailer that has a "doctor's office" on one side and a medical marijuana dispensary on the other. Bottom line, the "pot shop" situation in Colorado is just like the "pill mills" in the opioid crisis. *Kids can pay a few hundred bucks and get a medical marijuana card/fake prescription for some made-up ailment for the purpose of getting high.*

Pot doctors are churning out pricey "prescriptions" (which are just recommendations), just like the opioid clinics. You're supposed to have a bona fide relationship with your doctor, but not in this case. You only have to see the doctor annually to get your card renewed. Whoever sold my perfectly healthy son a marijuana card is basically a dope dealer in a white lab coat—a criminal physician who sold my son the ability to buy shatter at 18 years old and destroy his mind.

I am *not* talking about the majority of doctors, mind you. Most do not approve med cards; however, some "doctors" are little more than drug salespeople. Plus, there should be tracking of these controlled substances as we now have with opioids. They are just replicating pill mills and creating more addicts. It's easy–fill out the paperwork, pay the taxes, and open a clinic. They've sworn to do no harm, yet here are doctors giving marijuana to children with immature brains.

It's a very similar situation to the Netflix show "The Pharmacist." In the show, Dr. Cleggett was negligently prescribing opioids to young patients who claimed various maladies. How many teens have chronic pain at 18 years old? Johnny lied and said he had migraines (what teens tell each other to say) because there's no way to prove it—your pain is what you say it is. In the show, the pharmacist Dan Schneider said of his son, "Danny had talked to me about marijuana, saying it was safe and saying, 'But, Dad, I wouldn't go any further.' But every person goes further. Do you think any of them think it's going to lead to death or jail?" His son Danny was later murdered while attempting to purchase crack.

One of Johnny's Ambassadors Advisory Council members, Sally Schindel, also lost her dear son Andy to suicide. Andy told her he was coached (Sally's not sure if it was by friends, a dealer, or his med pot shop) on buying large quantities at the lowest per-ounce prices, then he'd sell small quantities at high prices to recoup his "investment."

Fairly predictably, without us monitoring him, Johnny went downhill. We know from a video that he tried cocaine, and he admitted to his therapist that he also tried LSD. In fact, a significant number of adolescents who experiment with marijuana try other drugs, too. According to the authors of the study "Cannabis as a Gateway Drug for Opioid Use Disorder,"[55] adolescent and young adult (through age 24) brain development is key to executive functioning and behavioral control. They note that cannabis can change adolescent gene expression and alter these key periods of neurodevelopment. Also, genes can predict the priming impact of cannabis on opioids, and there's likely individual variation in the risk of cannabis use in adolescence. It can have a negative effect on adolescent brain maturation and downstream vulnerability to opioid exposure and addiction.

Johnny stopped going to school altogether. His counselor and I stayed in close contact about what he needed to do to graduate, and I would nag him about it. I sometimes got him to turn in assignments, reminding him he had a scholarship on the line and nowhere else to go except rehab.

He still texted me several times a day about "mom" stuff and told me, "Adulting is hard." We would invite him to dinner periodically to check in with him and feed him a homecooked meal.

One night, he made a big announcement, "I just love marijuana. I'm going to smoke marijuana for the rest of my life!"

John repeated our party line, "Son, that is going to come back to bite you. It's not good for your brain."

I decided to try another tact, "Sweetie, why do you use marijuana?"

Johnny was confused, "What do you mean why?"

"Exactly what I said. Why do you use marijuana?"

He blinked and thought for a few minutes, "It makes me feel good, and I start feeling bad when I'm not, so it helps me."

I pressed the issue, "Okay, but besides feeling good, what is it about marijuana that you love so much?"

He looked thoughtful, "I guess it's about having a built-in circle of friends. It's about being accepted, you know? It's a social ritual. You automatically have people who do the same thing."

Ah, so using marijuana was no longer about feeling good. He had to use marijuana just to keep from feeling bad, a classic sign of substance use disorder. I felt so sad for him. I found out through our son James that Johnny had lost his "real" friends due to the choices he was making. Almost none of them were on speaking terms any longer, so he had to create new "friends" whose only connection was smoking weed together. It was the only way he felt like he belonged.

I asked him repeatedly to let me help him stop the marijuana, but he would say, "Mom, I'm fine. Leave me alone."

He wasn't fine. Someone texted a tip about him at school a couple of weeks later. That's a secret hotline used to report an infraction by a fellow student. The police were called, and his car, backpack, and locker were searched. He was suspended for five days from Monday, March 26 through Friday, March 30, 2018, for having Juuls, marijuana, and alcohol in his car. It was really five days of vacation.

Instead of being kicked off the property for five days, he should have had to go through a drug prevention class. Teens who violate drug policies should have to stay under surveillance at school and be educated, not given a free ride. We certainly wished a program like that would have been available for Johnny, like we created at Johnny's Ambassadors (*https://johnnysambassadors.org/ curriculum*). The officer who searched his car gave him a Minor in Possession (MIP) charge which put him in legal trouble again. Johnny told the officer he was legal for marijuana but couldn't produce his med card at that moment. The officer told him to bring in the med card to the sheriff's office that day. He never did get a citation for the marijuana, so I assume he was able to produce it.

Johnny asked me to help him schedule the MIP classes. I probably shouldn't have, but I helped him enroll and get through the MADD Impact Panel classes, Level 1 Alcohol classes, and eight hours of community service. Added to his curfew violation, reckless driving from the accident, a speeding ticket, and running a stop sign, he was just one error away from losing his driver's license.

May 1, 2018 — Can't Make Rent

I think Johnny forgot I had access to his bank account. I monitored his purchases and watched him spend his $5,000 in purchases at gas stations, for vape (before the law was changed to 21), lots of ATM withdrawals (cash for marijuana dispensaries), Venmo (likely drugs to sell), food (expensive eating out at restaurants), and pipe/tobacco shops (bongs, pens, rigs, pipes, etc.). He paid for his March and April rent, but by May, he was out of money.

May rent was due, and he asked me to come over to his house to talk. I parked my car, and we sat in the front seat of his car. I assume he didn't want me to come into his room to see his operation.

"Mom, I have the money, but it's not in cash form. I just need to convert it, but I'm going to need you to float me the money to pay my rent until I have it."

"No way, Johnny. You're 18, and you signed a lease. You spent your money on marijuana, pipe shops, and Lord knows what else, so you're going to need to work it out with your landlord."

"I already asked him for an extension. He's not going to give me a break and will charge me a penalty if I'm late."

"Then I recommend you get a job. I am not going to cover for your bad decision to sell drugs."

He was furious with me and called me every name in the book, which I won't repeat here.

"Son, I grieve your choices but will always love you and want to help you get better."

"That's a lie. You don't want to help me because you won't pay my rent. And how do you know what I'm buying?"

His eyes opened wide with realization, and the next day, he opened a separate checking account.

That night, the phone rang. It was Johnny calling from downtown Denver in a panic. He said a female friend from high school "stole his backpack" with all his "merchandise" inside. They had an argument, and she told him to get out of her car. He refused, so she called the police. He didn't want to tell the police his backpack was in her car with drugs in it, so she and her friend took off in the car with his backpack in the trunk. The problem was his school and personal items were also in the backpack.

Johnny gave us the home address of the girl. John and I drove to the house, knocked, and talked to the father about the situation. He went inside and came back with the backpack. We thanked him and left. Inside, we found his personal items (sunglasses, calculator, shirt, hat, etc.) and school items from the backpack, but there was nothing else. We found out later from Johnny that she sold the marijuana to one of her friends in exchange for a new Juul kit. The dad, of course, had no idea what was going on. Johnny couldn't exactly go to the police to accuse someone of stealing his drugs, so now he was broke. Welcome to drug dealing.

Johnny started calling me constantly to demand money. Sometimes, when I answered, he would simply scream, "F-YOU, Mom!" and hang up. It was absolutely heartbreaking.

His school counselor called me to say that if Johnny didn't take his English final, he would not earn the D he needed to graduate. I passed along the message to Johnny days in advance. I called him the night before to remind him and tell him to get a good night's sleep. I went over to his house the morning of his final, figuring he would oversleep, and knocked on his bedroom window (the one he was selling the marijuana out of). He was high as a kite. I was livid.

"Johnny, I am not leaving without you. I am very serious. Get up, put some clothes on, and come with me to school. You will put your butt in the chair and take your English final. If you don't, I will knock on the front door and wake your landlord up and make a scene. I've worked too hard to raise you for you not to graduate. You owe me this much. *Get out here now!*"

He did exactly as I said and came with me. I dropped him off at school for the last time, and he marched to the front door, hands stuffed in his pockets.

On May 16, 2018, Johnny graduated from high school. I was worried he would cause a scene, so John and Meagan attended the event, and I watched his graduation on the live stream. Johnny marched across the stage with his honor cords flowing, looking happy with a smile on his face. Except for his long hair which was unkempt and clearly hadn't been cut in many months, you wouldn't know he was a marijuana addict.

We asked friends and family to please not give him money for graduation. If they wanted to give him a gift, we said he needed food and Target gift cards. He was angry about that.

May 21, 2018 — Steals Our Dog

Three weeks into May, he still hadn't figured out a way to pay the rent. Johnny came to the house while we weren't at home, but his brother James was. He knocked on the door, and James opened it to see what he wanted. Johnny simply opened the second screen door and whistled to our dog, Lily. She ran toward him, excitedly, as she hadn't seen him for a while. James, not thinking anything of it, let her romp on the front porch with him for a minute. Suddenly, Johnny said, "Lily, come," and he turned and ran toward his car. Lily followed obediently behind (she's an Australian Shepherd). He opened the car door, she jumped in, and he drove off. James stood on the porch, stunned, and watched them drive away. Panicked, he called me and said, "Johnny just stole Lily!"

We rushed home, and John received this text from him, "It's my dog, and you're giving me that money. Call the police, and I'll fight you in court if I have to. You're not getting my dog back, so it's either that or you're never seeing me again. You don't want the police involved with me. Give me my f***ing money. I worked my ass off to graduate for your f***ing b***ch of a wife, and she's not going to give me it. If you call the police on me, I'm never forgiving you. You're already treading on pretty thin ice as it is. You know what? Call the police. If I see a single cop at my door, you won't like the result. You want your dog back, John?"

John went over and took the dog back, of course. Johnny promised he would pay us back every penny, so I paid rent directly to Shawn after that to ensure Johnny wasn't handling any money. I know, I know ... I shouldn't have paid his rent. But I am his mother, and I just couldn't bear the thought of him living on the street. Being so sick and addicted, he was bound to get in even more trouble. Little did I know.

May 24, 2018 — Criminal Mischief

Just a few days later, Johnny received a call from a friend (a young woman). She reportedly told him she felt unsafe with the person she was with, and he wouldn't let her leave the house. She texted Johnny that she feared for her safety and was afraid of being raped. So, Johnny got the address of where she was, drove over there, and threw a rock through the glass window over their front door. When I asked him later what he was thinking, he said, "Um, well, I really wasn't. I thought it would get the attention of her parents." Boy, did it ever! The father sued Johnny for criminal mischief. Johnny asked me to help him navigate the court process. Why I agreed to help him, I don't know, but we wound up in court several times to answer for his vandalism.

One morning, I picked him up at his house to drive him to the courthouse to plead his case. As we were driving, I told him, "I want you to know that no matter what you're involved in, there is nothing you can do to make me stop loving you." He became angry. He said, "Oh, yes there is!" and started a tirade of verbal abuse. We arrived at the courthouse and pulled into a parking spot.

We got out of the car with Johnny still yelling profanities at me and blaming me for everything that happened to him. As we walked toward the front door, I said, "You might want to calm down now because you're making a scene in front of a courthouse." He retorted, "I'll do whatever the hell I want, b***h," and he shoved me on the shoulders, hard. I stumbled backward and caught myself before I fell. While this was happening, a taxi was pulling up, apparently to pick someone up. The driver saw what was happening and pulled over to the curb. He got out and started to approach us. "Hey, you there!" he yelled at Johnny. I quickly told him, "It's okay. This is my son." He stopped and stared at me with the saddest look in his eyes. He turned and walked back to his car.

We went inside, and Johnny proceeded to plead his case. He was told that if he fixed the window, the owner of the house would drop the charges. On the way home, Johnny said he was hungry and asked if we could stop by Chick-fil-A. We ate our food in silence in the parking lot. I couldn't think of a single thing to say to my son. Then Johnny said, "Dad told me never to put my hands on you again, and I'm sorry. I don't want you to be afraid of me." I looked at him sadly and simply said, "Like I said, there is nothing you can do to make me stop loving you."

I thought the legal trouble would end there, but sadly, it didn't. In June, the "Bad News Girlfriend" entered the scene. For ease, from here forward, I will refer to her as BNG. Johnny met a young woman through his marijuana "friends." He told me she was mentally ill with bipolar disorder and borderline personality disorder. She was on medications and used daily dabs to "control it," so obviously, it wasn't under control. They quickly developed a codependent relationship. She used sex to get what she wanted from him and try to make him love her. After he died, I could read the texts between them and see the photos on his phone. They confirmed she was a very sick young woman.

A couple weeks before Johnny died, here is how he described BNG in his journal, "What you have to understand about (BNG) is that she's extremely mentally unstable because of her BPD and takes concentrated dabs of marijuana throughout every single day, which only worsens her condition. She self-harms a lot, and during an argument last year, slit her wrist open in an attempt to 'win.' She always uses impulsive, self-destructive behaviors with no thought of the consequences. She has very unstable relationships with everyone. She has explosive anger and extreme mood swings, often catching you off guard when it seemed one minute everything was going fine. For (BNG), every day is variable with who she's going to be, how she's going to act, and which side of her is going to come out. She constantly fears abandonment and will do ANYTHING to hold on to her relationships, including physically or mentally abusing and harming the people around her, including her family. As her ultimate move, she would say she was going to kill herself to get her way."

One night, they were out with two other friends. As he described in his journal, they were in a public area, and she "had a manic episode and started screaming at the top of her lungs and smashed her head against a brick wall...someone called the police...she slapped me in the face...went to jail." Obviously, they broke up after this. BNG was charged with domestic violence, and he had to go to court. She was sentenced to one year of diversion with classes and agreed not to harass or intimidate Johnny. I hoped that would be the end of her and the end of his legal troubles. But sadly, it wasn't.

One of Johnny's friends told him his Toyota Camry needed some antifreeze and offered to take care of it while he went to work. So, Johnny gave him his car to get that accomplished. The friend promptly drove to Walmart and stole the antifreeze from the store. The parking lot cameras captured the friend getting into Johnny's car with the stolen antifreeze. The police were given the footage, and they looked up the license plate from the camera. The car was titled in my husband's name, not Johnny's. The front doorbell rang, and a police officer stood there.

"John Stack?"

My husband is used to this name confusion, "Which one?"

"Your son stole an item from Walmart about an hour ago."

"I'm confused because I talked to him while he was at work around that time."

The officer took out his phone, showed John the photo of the other boy, and said, "The parking camera caught him."

"That's not my son. He must have loaned his car to that boy."

"Well, now he's wanted for shoplifting. Can you put me in touch with your son?"

The officer called Johnny who agreed to meet the officer at a nearby park. The officer drove over, and since it was an active investigation, they towed and impounded Johnny's car. Well, this was an interesting situation. With Johnny about to go off to college, John and I were talking about how it would be better to leave his car here. Colorado State University had great transportation options for students, and most freshmen didn't take cars up there. They simply walked, biked, or took the free shuttle around campus. Perhaps not having a car or money would keep him on campus and out of trouble. When the officer called John to give him an update, John told the officer that since he owned the title, he didn't want Johnny to have the car back. So, the officer stalled for us. The police impounded the car until it was time for Johnny to leave for college.

CHAPTER 4:

THE BREAK

August 14, 2018 — Trashes His Room

It was finally time to go to Colorado State University (CSU). We helped Johnny move his belongings out of his rental house. He needed to get unpacked and re-packed for his new dorm room, so he was to spend one night in his old bedroom. When we arrived home, he walked upstairs to his room and immediately became violent. He trashed his room and destroyed many of his childhood possessions. I stood outside the door helplessly, crying and begging him to please stop. John kept his distance with a watchful eye, so Johnny didn't become physical with me. Johnny ripped apart trophies, smashed photo frames, and tore the head off a bobblehead I had made of him one Christmas. He pulled all his books off his bookshelf and threw souvenirs against the wall. When he was done, he stormed past me, went into his bathroom, and proceeded to trash that, too. When he was done, he moved down the hall to James' room. James stood his ground in his doorway. Johnny must have realized his younger brother was larger, heavier, and stronger, because when James pointedly said, "Stop," Johnny stopped. He went back into his bedroom and crumpled to the floor. I went to him, and he let me rub his back and talk softly to him. With a heavy heart, I cleaned up the mess and put back what could be saved.

I didn't sleep a wink all night long. I kept picturing Johnny coming into my bedroom with a knife. He acted like he hated me so much, but I kept reminding myself that was the marijuana, not my son. We had a lock on the handle of our bedroom door, but it wasn't a great one. A few days later, John installed locks on our door and James' bedroom door. We knew we were no longer safe sleeping in our own bedrooms when Johnny was home on break. The marijuana had made him dangerous.

August 15, 2018 — University #1

We drove Johnny up to CSU the next morning and moved him into his dorm. Freshman orientation started that evening. He was so sour and foul and wouldn't even let me touch his items without permission, so the move-in process took a very long time. Then, his new roommate arrived (who will go nameless to protect his identity as will all of the young people in this story). The roommate's parents made small talk with us while he arranged his possessions. They told us they were from Minnesota.

Johnny and the roommate took off alone. John and I sort of wandered around while most students hung out with their folks at the carnival. We finally saw him and went to say goodbye. He barely acknowledged us, so we left to drive home. Later that night, I called Johnny and said, "Hey, I didn't see you much, but I'm glad you and (roommate) hit it off. I'm just calling to wish you luck and tell you I love you." Johnny said, "Yes, (roommate) and I hung out on the oval and smoked weed." I was pretty angry he would say something like that to throw it in my face after everything we'd done to get him there. I thought, "How in the world did he get a hold of it that quickly?" (This was before I knew he had a med card.)

Over the next couple of weeks, we connected every other day or so when he needed something. He told me he was figuring out how to get around on campus and was glad we brought his bike up there. He went to his classes and participated in some activities, so I thought perhaps everything would be okay.

August 30, 2018 — Suicidal Text

It wasn't. Two weeks later on August 30, 2018, I received a very chilling text from Johnny about 10:00 p.m. that said, "I'm having a hard time meeting people." I texted back reassuringly, "It's normal to feel worried about making new friends, but you will!" Johnny replied, "Is it normal to think about killing myself every day?"

That text started the worst 14 months of my life and ended with the worst day of my life on November 20, 2019, when Johnny completed suicide. Our grief continues to this day, and I imagine it always will.

At that time, our then-23-year-old daughter Meagan lived farther north than we did, between Denver and Fort Collins. So, I called her and told her what Johnny said. I said, "Sweetie, this is going to be hard, but I need you to go get him. I don't care what you say but just get him to go with you to your house. He is much more likely to go with you than me." She told him she was surprising him with a trip to the CSU versus CU Rocky Mountain Showdown football game the next day, so he went with her willingly. They got back to her house around midnight. Meagan told us that while they were driving, Johnny talked about his ideations of jumping off a building.

Very early the next morning, John and I drove up to Meagan's house. We waited for Johnny to wake up and were sitting in her living room when he walked in. He broke down in sobs, and he let me hold him. I told him I was so worried about him, and we needed to get him some help. I asked him to voluntarily agree to be evaluated at a mental hospital. "And if I don't agree?" Johnny asked. "Then I will call the police, and they will forcibly take you. Then you will end up at a facility that isn't near our house, and I won't be close enough to be able to help you as much." He looked at Meagan and said, "You lied to me." I jumped in, "I told her to. It's not her fault." After much conversation, hugs, and crying, Johnny agreed to go to the mental hospital.

August 31, 2018 — First Mental Hospital

We said goodbye to Meagan who had acted bravely through it all. To this day, she still feels bad about fibbing to him, but she knows how important it was to get him to her house and safe. John,

Johnny, and I got in our car and drove to a mental hospital called Denver Springs in Englewood, Colorado, about 10 minutes from our home. I had already talked with the intake staff about the procedure the night before. It was a walk-in hospital, much like an emergency room. During the drive, we talked about his feelings, and Johnny admitted, "(Roommate's name) and I have been pretty much dabbing non-stop since we got there a couple weeks ago." I said, "What do you mean by dabbing?" "Marijuana, Mom," he said. At the time, I didn't understand the connection between suicidal thinking and marijuana.

Negative Effects of Cannabis

The evidence-based negative effects of cannabis on adolescents are many and varied,[56] especially for young people.[57] Two independent studies of adolescents who use marijuana have demonstrated a big elevation in suicide attempts:

1) The first study[58] was a large longitudinal study of over 2,000 adolescents conducted in Australia and New Zealand. It found that teens who are daily users of marijuana before age 17 had a seven-fold increase in suicide attempts compared to non-users.

2) The second study[59] was conducted with 700 teens and corrected for a prior history of depression or other mood disorders. In other words, they factored out kids who were already depressed when they started using marijuana. They found that marijuana use in those who weren't previously depressed increased the risk of a suicide attempt 7.5-fold.

There is also evidence that marijuana's effect can be more immediate.[60] This comes from a recent study illustrating the likelihood of suicidal thoughts increasing on the days an adolescent uses marijuana.

Johnny became just one of the 80 youths in Colorado ages 15-19 who died by suicide in 2019. According to the Colorado Department of Public Health and Environment, in 2019, suicide was the #1 cause of death for adolescents ages 10-19. In Colorado, the THC-positive toxicology screens in youth ages 15-19 have consistently increased over the past several years (while such data was being collected by the Colorado Department of Health) such that THC became the leading drug found in suicide victims of that age range.[61] (It noted that over 36% of youth who died by suicide were positive for THC in 2018, the last year data is available.) That figure doesn't include those young people like Johnny who had *no* THC in their systems at the time but were psychotic from previous marijuana use and where a toxicology test wasn't ordered.

It's no coincidence that the increases in suicides and toxicology rates with THC in Colorado teens are correlated. As a mother, I want the world to know my son isn't just a statistic. He mattered. There *is a reason Johnny died*—and it is marijuana. Johnny didn't have any delusions before marijuana. Johnny's marijuana use led to changes in his brain development[62] which led to mental illness which led to suicide. So, while it's rare to die from an acute overdose of THC, we know for a fact that long-term cannabis use can result in thoughts of suicide[63] and suicide itself.

To analyze the science on marijuana and suicide and its causal relationship, neuroscientist Christine L. Miller, Ph.D., wrote a white paper for Johnny's Ambassadors[64] in September 2020 titled "Applying the Bradford Hill Criteria for Causation to the Relationship Between Marijuana Use and Suicidal Behavior." As Miller wrote, "In 1965, Sir Bradford Hill developed a set of tests designed to elucidate causal relationships in epidemiology. These criteria have subsequently become accepted as important standards for epidemiological and clinical science."

There are nine Bradford Hill Criteria:

1) Demonstration of a strong association between the causative agent and the outcome

2) Consistency of the findings across research sites and methodologies

3) Demonstration of specificity of the causative agent in terms of the outcomes it produces (not applicable in this illustration)

4) Demonstration of the appropriate temporal sequence so that the causative agent occurs prior to the outcome

5) Demonstration of a biological gradient in which more of the causative agent leads to a poorer outcome

6) Demonstration of a biologic rationale such that it makes sense that the suspected agent causes the outcome

7) Coherence of the findings such that the causation argument is in agreement with what we already know

8) Experimental evidence

9) Evidence from analogous conditions (not applicable in this illustration)

Miller concluded that all except #4 in this list apply to the relationship between marijuana and suicidal behavior, not just suicidal thought. (For that single criterion, not enough evidence has been presented to prove an appropriate temporal sequence, though Miller pointed out that the data are "strongly suggestive.")

Ultimately, she made it clear, "*The weight of the current evidence should be regarded as strong enough to elicit widespread public health warnings about the suspected role of marijuana use in precipitating suicidal behaviors, since the mandate of the relevant authorities is to err on the side of protecting public health rather than to establish scientific certainty beyond a shadow of a doubt.*"

That's as close to a ringing declaration that marijuana use can lead to suicidal ideation and suicide as we have thus far. I have little doubt that within the next few years, that link will be proven beyond a scientific doubt. By then, we will have lost many generations of young people. How long did it take for them to make the connection between tobacco use and death?

When we arrived at Denver Springs, Johnny was asked to fill out some paperwork. One form asked, "Are you having thoughts of harming yourself?" He checked, "Yes." I breathed a sigh of relief because I knew (and he didn't) that walking through that door with the "Yes" box checked resulted in an M1 Hold for 72 hours. (An M1 Hold is placed when an individual is deemed to be in imminent danger of harming him or herself.)

The nurse called him, and he was in the exam room for about 30 minutes. I started to wonder what was going on when the door opened, and the nurse motioned for me to come back. Johnny was being difficult and defiant and refused to stay there. She asked me to try to convince him to stay willingly. After some conversation, he suddenly stood up and tried to walk out the door, which was locked, of course.

He whirled around and glared at me, "So, I'm a prisoner here?"

"Honey, please let them try to help you."

After another hour of back and forth, he finally let them lead him down the hall. At the end of the hall, he turned around and looked back at me one more time. I gave him a thumbs-up then burst into tears as he walked out of view.

The next day, we brought over the items he could have, such as shoes without shoelaces, sweatshirts without strings, sweatpants without ties, playing cards, and books. We were upset to learn that since it was Labor Day weekend, there would be no doctors on duty for a couple of days. How were they supposed to diagnose him, get him medicine if needed, and monitor him within his mandatory hold of 72 hours?

During visiting hours, we could see him briefly in a little room, and we could talk on the phone a couple of times a day. On one phone call, Johnny told me, "I'm just going to kill myself when I get out of here anyway." I immediately called and reported what he said to the case worker and begged her not to let the doctors release him. He finally got to see a doctor on the fourth day. The doctor prescribed Wellbutrin. Then they advised me Johnny said he no longer felt suicidal, so they were not going to be able to hold him. "What?!" I yelled. "You're going to give him a new medicine, let him lie to you, and let him out of there still suicidal?" I was told there was nothing they could do legally because he was 18.

On his discharge paperwork, the doctor wrote Johnny's diagnosis: THC ABUSE SEVERE.

THC Abuse Severe

So, yes, if you doubt it, it's true that people can feel suicidal after using marijuana, especially when they are young and use high-potency products with high frequency. I know because it happened to my son in front of my very eyes.

We took Johnny home, and he was agitated. We had conversations about his next step, and he said he couldn't concentrate and do well in school. We agreed that now probably wasn't the best time for him to have the added pressure of school, and he should focus on getting himself well again. I promised he could try again in the spring, and with all his AP credits, it wouldn't set him back a bit. He agreed to disenroll from CSU and submitted his paperwork online. It was hugely disappointing to us all because he had worked so hard for the scholarship he was walking away from.

Once a student disenrolls, he or she must move items out of the dorm to stop paying room and board. We planned to go back up to the dorm to retrieve all of his belongings the next day. The next morning, Johnny said he was tired and asked if he could just stay home and sleep longer, so John and I agreed and drove up to bring his things home.

In his room, we came across a box in his desk drawer that had the words "Nectar Collector Kit" printed on top. "Hmmm, that's odd, I wonder what this is?" I thought. I opened it, and there was a strange brownish sticky substance I'd never seen before. It looked like a big ball of nasty earwax.

"What is this?" I thought. I showed it to John and asked, "What *is* this stuff?" John didn't know either.

I walked over to his roommate who sat on his bed the entire time, staring at us without so much as lifting a finger. "What is this?" I asked him. He shrugged and said, "Dabs." Ohhhh, ding ding. That was my first introduction to marijuana concentrates.

As we were in the car about to pull away, my cell phone rang. It was Johnny.

"Hello, love. We're on our way home."

I will never forget the cold dagger I felt in my heart when I heard Johnny shrieking. *"Mom, I just tried to kill myself."*

"WHAT?! Johnny, what have you done? Did you take pills? What did you do?" I didn't know whether I needed to get him medical attention right away.

"I tried to hang myself in my bedroom closet. It didn't work."

"Where are you now?"

"I'm at home."

"Stay right there. Here, talk to Dad for a minute."

I gave John my phone and called the police on John's phone. I reported what happened, told them we were 75 minutes away, and begged them to go check on my son. I gave the phone back to John to stay on the line with the police. I was able to keep Johnny talking to me on the phone for about ten minutes as I tried to comfort him.

Then Johnny heard John talking to the police, "Who is Dad talking to? You didn't call the police, did you?"

"Johnny, please let us help you. Please don't do anything to hurt yourself. Talk to me!"

Through Johnny's phone, I heard the garage door opening, and Johnny hung up on me.

"Johnny! Johnny, no!" I wailed as I dialed again, trying to get him back on the phone. I have never been so scared or felt so helpless in all my life.

Right then, thank God, the dispatcher told John they had him. Johnny was pulling out of our driveway when the police drove down our street. They blocked his car with their vehicles and prevented him from driving away. The police officer confirmed to dispatch that Johnny had rope burns on his neck. They handcuffed him and took him to the emergency room at Skyridge Hospital nearby to be evaluated. I explained to the dispatcher that he had just been released from Denver Springs for suicidal thinking. I asked her to please ensure he was taken back there after they examined him. Before we hung up, the dispatcher advised me his car was left in the street. I called my best friend and asked her to go into the house, get the spare keys, and move it into the driveway.

We drove as fast as safely possible and arrived at the hospital.

"Oh, Johnny!" I cried as I rushed into his room in the ER. I reached for him, and he rebuffed me.

"Leave me alone!"

Johnny ignored me while I quietly cried, and John stood stoically by his side. I was so relieved he was still alive. I can't explain the feeling of almost losing your child and then not losing him. I felt desperate to help him but didn't know how. They checked him out, and he was physically fine with no damage to his neck.

Then the ER doctor came over to talk to us. He had spoken to the doctor at Denver Springs who advised him of Johnny's THC levels. The doctor explained it can take weeks for the marijuana to exit his body. He would need to be detained until then, and Denver Springs had agreed to take him back. Because he had attempted suicide, he didn't have a choice about staying. They were concerned he might be violent, so he was put in cuffs and taken back in a waiting ambulance.

Right away, we started looking up the Nectar Kit and researching marijuana concentrates. We watched videos of people dabbing and making shatter at home. And we were shocked by what we found!

If you haven't used marijuana in five years, you have no idea what it's like today. I recommend you read the original guest blog post written for Johnny's Ambassadors by Ben Cort titled "You Know Nothing About Weed" *(https://johnnysambassadors.org/about-weed)*. The research we read about the harms of high-potency marijuana on the developing mind was startling. To date, there exists over 35,000 articles on marijuana research in the National Institutes of Health's National Library of Medicine *(ncbi.nlm.nih.gov/?term=marijuana)*. The pro-pot industry can't refute these proven studies.

Weeks later, the marijuana wore off, and the Wellbutrin started to help. Johnny was sober and no longer felt suicidal. No longer antagonistic, he was rather sullen and depressed from dropping out of school and losing his scholarship. He had developed a habit of pulling his hair. We visited him each day and participated in joint family counseling and activity sessions as well as one-on-one counseling. During this process, we asked for his agreement not to use marijuana if he were to return home, and he agreed. So, under the condition that he attend an Intensive Outpatient Program (IOP) at Denver Springs for 14 days, they released him to our care.

September 12, 2018 — Finding Treatment

We dropped Johnny off for the first day of his IOP. When I went to pick him up, the administrator called me back and asked me to pay for the day.

"Why? Won't you bill my insurance company for the complete program?"

"Johnny checked himself out of the program today, so we already called your insurance company and would like to collect your co-insurance."

"WHAT?! How is that possible? He agreed as a condition of release just yesterday that he would participate in this program!"

"Once they leave here, there is nothing we can do. He's an adult and can release himself when he's not in the hospital."

It was unbelievable he could do that. I was fuming when Johnny came down the hall.

"What is this all about, Johnny? Why did you check yourself out?"

"It was stupid. They had me drawing pictures of myself and listening to some clown, and I didn't like the other people there. I'd rather do something else."

I shook my head, feeling at a complete loss. *Now what am I supposed to do?* I thought. *He just tried to kill himself a few weeks ago, and here he is in my care.*

So, I called my insurance company, Cigna, to find out who they recommended he see. They gave me a list of mental health programs, and I started making phone calls. At the time, I didn't know to do my own research first to see what was out there. (To help you, we have listed several locator services on our website at *https://johnnysambassadors.org/parents*.) It was tricky finding someone who took 18-year-olds because they couldn't be with the youth and weren't old enough for the 21+ programs.

Our first attempt was a center called Sandstone Care. It took about 40 minutes in rush hour traffic to get there. People at the center seemed disorganized, and there were young kids running all over the place. Johnny was the oldest one there. We did the intake, and then the director said he had to be drug tested. He wasn't mentally prepared to provide a sample, so that was difficult for him. I left, knowing this wasn't going to go well. Sure enough, he refused to be part of that "kids program" when I picked him up.

Next, they tried putting him in an older group. I picked him up afterward, and he was sullen. I asked how it went, and he said, "Well, Mom, those a**holes basically made fun of me. They are all hooked on heroin and meth, and they made me feel weak that I'm only addicted to marijuana." Poor kid. My heart broke for him. Here he was trying to get help, and these mean people didn't understand the risk and harm of marijuana addiction. Understandably, he disliked that group therapy as well, and there were no additional options for us there. I received the following discharge letter:

September 25, 2018

To Whom It May Concern,

I am writing this letter to inform you that Johnny Stack completed a Clinical Assessment at Sandstone Care, in Denver, CO. Sandstone Care is a licensed treatment facility offering intensive outpatient services to clients who are recovering from co-occurring disorders or substance abuse and mental illness.

Johnny presented to Sandstone Care on 9/18/18, after a turnaround admission to Denver Springs for SI — attempt. At the time of his assessment, he had spent a total of 14 days with Denver Springs, 09/01/18 — 09/05/18 — 09/12/18.

He presented with cannabis use, social phobia, as well as Major Depressive d/o — Dysthymia. (Laura's note: Dysthymia is defined as having depressed mood most of the time along with two of the following symptoms: poor appetite or overeating, insomnia or excessive sleep, low energy or fatigue, low self-esteem, poor concentration or indecisiveness, and hopelessness.) Johnny was assessed as appropriate for YA IOP (young adult intensive outpatient program) and presented for an intake on 9/20/18. During the time that Johnny was in group, he reported that his anxiety became unmanageable in a group setting. Johnny and his parents determined that a group setting was not the treatment intervention they wished to pursue.

It was this writer's impression that Johnny may benefit from dual-diagnosis programming to focus on how his mental health exacerbates his substance use and vice-versa.

So, following their recommendation, we tried to find dual-diagnosis programming and again looked at the recommendations from Cigna. I called the admissions counselor at the place on the list named Palmer Lake Recovery Village. He told me that since Johnny was "only addicted to marijuana," he knew Cigna wouldn't pay for it. He suggested Johnny should "list something else he was addicted to like LSD" on the application. I told him I didn't think my son would go for that. Sure enough, Johnny was angry and refused. After Johnny's death, I got a call from a woman at Palmer Lake to "see how Johnny was doing" and "if they could help me." I had several choice words for the poor lady and feel bad about what I said. She was just doing her job.

There weren't any other centers listed, and it didn't dawn on us to send him out of state. No one suggested that, and after making so many phone calls, I just didn't know how to find help. It was difficult to find proper medical treatment for cannabis use disorder (CUD) and the mental illness that resulted.

An Excellent Resource

Crystal Collier, Ph.D., is on the Scientific Advisory Board for Johnny's Ambassadors. She offers a "Continuum of Care" in her book, *The NeuroWhereAbouts Guide: A Neurodevelopmental Guide for Parents and Families Who Want to Prevent Youth High-Risk Behavior*. It was written to help parents determine the most suitable treatment or intervention option depending on age, level of use, life stage, educational need, and stage of change. The goal is to keep your teen from moving from experimentation to misuse to abuse to dependence.

If the child is drug tested and doesn't stay sober, the next level of behavior modification is put into place, and the next level of treatment is implemented. She says drug testing should begin at age 11 or 12 at least once or twice a year. It is the #1 refusal skill your child will need at parties, "I'd love to, but my mom drug tests me." If you're suspicious or if your child is using, increase the frequency of testing. It's about putting boundaries into place, holding your child responsible for behaviors, and staying accountable to the consequences outlined. (You can watch her webinar in our previous Johnny's Ambassadors webinars at *www. JohnnysAmbassadors.org/recorded-webinars.*)

October 15, 2018 — Recovery

Next, I called a therapist friend for suggestions. He referred me to a psychiatrist who he said was one of the best in town. He turned out to be the worst person we could have picked. We didn't know it at the time, but he and the other female physician's assistant (whom I will refer to as the Psychiatric PA) didn't know about concentrates. The Psychiatric PA once texted me, "If he absolutely won't quit marijuana, have him switch strains from Sativa to something less stimulating such as Indica." I had to give *them* an education about dabbing based on what we found.

Good Lord, Johnny needed to be told to stop completely! Maybe if they had said, "Give it up for good," he might have changed directions at this point. I don't blame them though, but they certainly didn't help Johnny in that regard. Also, it's entirely possible Johnny wasn't honest with them about his usage because I wasn't welcome back in the office while they talked.

I believe it should be *mandatory* education that all healthcare professionals go through rudimentary training in marijuana, because these people were exactly like I used to be—clueless. In Colorado, the potency and products are completely limitless and unregulated, and it's certainly not the "weed" that voters approved in 2012.

I was hopeful this doctor could help him. On the intake form, I wrote, "Johnny's self-esteem is very low, and he is very negative about himself and his future. He doesn't know what he wants to do and feels incapable. He struggles with even very simple decisions. His anger and rages are currently not there, but he still seems very depressed. He is embarrassed about his red cheeks. The marijuana didn't help of course. He says he needs a brain scan as he has degenerative brain disease or a hole in his brain. He doesn't currently have any close friends, so we want to get him engaged in other activities and perhaps a college course locally..."

The doctor took Johnny off the Wellbutrin and put him on desvenlafaxine (Pristiq). He said it would improve his mood, feelings of well-being, and energy levels as well as restore the balance of serotonin and norepinephrine in his brain to reduce anxiety.

Okay, so we found a psychiatrist. What about a therapist? Johnny didn't want to go back to his old therapist, John. I believe it was because he felt ashamed and wanted John to remember him as he was. The psychiatrist recommended an anxiety treatment program in Denver and suggested Johnny get a job to keep himself occupied.

So, we talked with Johnny about what kind of job he would enjoy that would be therapeutic and not stressful to him. He said he would like to work around dogs. We worked on his résumé together and did some mock interviews. When he felt confident enough, he called a dog hospital and kennel just ten minutes from our house. Amazingly, they currently needed a kennel assistant. After a couple of interviews, he was hired. He really enjoyed that job and loved playing with the dogs.

But after his first day, he came home discouraged and said, "Mom, my brain is broken. I need a brain scan. I can't remember the simplest instructions, and I'm going to get fired."

"Your memory will improve now that you're off the marijuana. Just give it some time. It's going to be okay," was my response.

Johnny agreed to try the anxiety therapy program the psychiatrist recommended. It was with Dr. Michael Stein at Anxiety Solutions of Denver. He was in the program from October 25, 2018, to January 3, 2019, and it proved to be excellent for him. By the end, he felt comfortable striking up a random conversation with someone in the Cherry Creek mall. He found he could talk to anyone. His confidence was built, and the medicine seemed to be helping!

Johnny felt so good by early November that he wanted to go to school again. I was thrilled! He didn't want to go back to CSU due to embarrassment and his negative memories. So, we visited the University of Northern Colorado (UNC) in Greeley together, and he liked it. Since he had disenrolled at CSU after two weeks, UNC treated him as a new incoming freshman and gave him a scholarship for his grades and test scores! It was not as good as the first scholarship, but we were all pleased, nonetheless. So, it was all set—Johnny would go to UNC in January 2019. We all felt happy and hopeful.

Then unknown to us, toward the end of 2018, we discovered he had started sneaking out in the middle of the night to see an old buddy down the street who also used marijuana. John got an internet deal with Comcast that included a security system with an alarm on the back sliding door that leads into our backyard. We never set that alarm because I kept forgetting to turn it off in the morning when I let our dog Lily out. I woke up the household on more than one occasion.

One night, I awoke and felt hungry enough that I couldn't sleep. I padded softly downstairs so as not to wake up the guys. While I was in the kitchen munching on crackers, Johnny quietly came in through the back door! I almost scared him out of his mind just standing there, minding my own business.

Of course, he had every excuse in the book such as so-and-so was down and needed help, etc. I confronted him about using marijuana, and he swore up and down he was clean. I should have drug tested him as a condition of him living at home, but again, I wasn't aware that was an option. I don't blame his friend because he didn't know marijuana had caused Johnny so many mental health problems.

I told John what happened, and he checked the logs for the back door security system. Sure enough, Johnny had also snuck out on November 26 and three other days in December. We showed Johnny the logs. We asked him how he could possibly think of using marijuana again when he had just been in the mental hospital a few months before, knowing marijuana made him suicidal. And he was just getting better. Johnny continued to deny using it which we didn't believe for a second. I guess he couldn't resist the siren song. Maybe he thought he could handle it or that suicidal thoughts wouldn't happen again. At that point, we told him we would be alarming the system before we go to bed so he couldn't open any doors without us knowing.

After that, I had an uneasy feeling about him going away to college again. I wasn't sure it would be fine, but he really wanted to go.

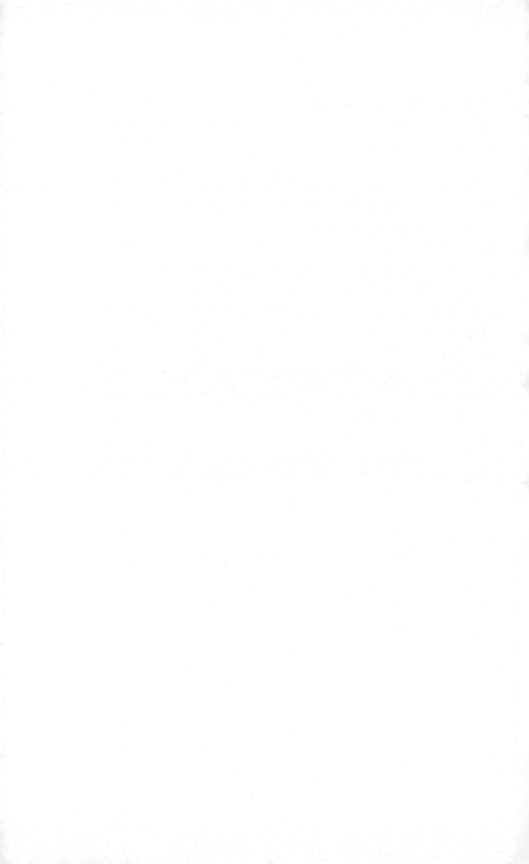

CHAPTER 5:

THE PSYCHOSIS

January 8, 2019 — University #2

We drove Johnny 90 minutes away to the University of Northern Colorado, feeling simultaneously eager and worried. Parking was cheap at UNC, so we let him have his own car. We wanted him to be able to get home quickly if he needed to. This time, he let me help him move into his dorm room at South Hall and clean it. We took photos of him in his new room—positive, confident, and smiling. I look at photos of myself wearing my "Mama Bear" shirt (UNC Bears) with his arm around my shoulders, and I remember the immense hope I had for my boy.

We drove away and left Johnny there with a hug and a "you've got this." We prayed he would be okay.

According to Johnny's reports and the hall director I connected with later, everything started off well. Johnny made friends and went to his classes. Then sadly, he gravitated toward the wrong crowd. He found a new girlfriend on his floor who dabbed and fell right back into marijuana use. His Snapchat photos show him partying and dabbing with friends. But of course, he didn't tell us. We visited him a few times, bought him supplies, and met his girlfriend. Everything seemed okay.

His friend (the one who also went to IdRaHaJe and UNC) later told me they would vape THC in his shower without the water running. She said, "You just put a towel under the door and turn on the bathroom fan. People don't know you're smoking. Johnny had a very high tolerance. He hit his dab pen all day throughout the day, like a Juul. He was basically high all the time. He would only let me take one hit from it because he said I would 'green out' and puke all over or have a really bad high."

April 5, 2019 —
Middle of the Night Break

My cell phone rang at 3:00 a.m. It was Johnny. I got up to leave the bedroom so I wouldn't wake John. I whispered loudly, "Johnny, what's wrong?"

"Mom, I found out my girlfriend was cheating on me with someone who claims to be my best friend, so I banged on her door just now and screamed at her. I bugged her computer. My dorm room is bugged, too."

"I'm so sorry that happened with your girlfriend, honey. What do you mean your dorm room is bugged?"

"Yes, and I'm going to need a new phone since the FBI is spying on me through my iPhone. They actually think I'm a terrorist."

"What in the world are you talking about, Johnny?"

"I'll tell you more about it tomorrow. I've got to get some sleep," and he hung up. It was the middle of the night, and I thought my son had just literally lost his mind. I had no idea what to do.

A few hours later, my phone rang with a number I didn't recognize. I answered, "Hello?" It was Johnny.

"Hi, Mom, it's me. Okay, actually, it's not true I bugged her computer. I was just saying that."

"Johnny, where are you calling from? What number is this?"

"It's a burner phone I bought at Target."

"What? Wait, why would you lie to me about bugging your girlfriend's computer?"

"Mom, you know why. Since my dorm room is bugged, they were listening to me, so I wanted to worry them with my power."

"Who do you mean by 'they' are listening, Johnny?"

"Mom, you know."

"Know what?"

Johnny hung up on me. I started calling everyone I could think of at the university. No one would help me or tell me anything because of their "privacy" laws! My kid is acting bizarre, and no one will tell me what's happening because he's over 18? This was outrageous! Can't they tell he's lost it? Apparently, because he had made such a scene, the hall director and student services called him in for a meeting. Unknown to me, they switched his dorm room to North Hall because it wasn't bugged! Seriously?

I learned that no one called the police. No one had him admitted to a mental hospital for a psych evaluation because they believed he wasn't a danger to himself. They kept telling me they were "handling" it. Perhaps I should have sued them. After his death, I talked to his residential advisor (RA) on his floor who told me he *did* tell her he felt like killing himself. But instead of reporting it, she talked to him about Jesus, which I appreciate, but he still needed help!

I kept calling Johnny, but his phone was going straight to voicemail. I called the other phone, but voicemail wasn't set up. I left messages and emails, asking him to please come home and let us help him. We couldn't just drive up there and forcibly make him leave. We didn't have a key to his room or know where he was. I wasn't even sure if *he* knew he was having a mental break. I did know he did not want to go to the mental hospital again.

Facts About Psychosis

This was the first time Johnny ever exhibited any kind of psychosis. Before, it was suicidal thinking. But with repeated assaults on the brain, marijuana can *cause* psychosis. Many people scoff at the notion that the relationship is causal, but they haven't read the newest research. Those at the forefront of such studies were eventually convinced that the association was causal. [65] Researchers first needed to determine which came first, the marijuana use or the psychosis.[66] The consensus is that use of marijuana with a THC content[67] over 10% increases the risk of a psychotic disorder four- to five-fold.[68]

Dr. Erik Messamore defines psychosis as "a neurological symptom related to misperception. Our brains make perception errors all the time. Psychosis happens when the misperceptions happen often enough that the conscious mind begins to make sense of them by forming unusual beliefs. If my brain starts to misperceive as highly significant things that are ordinary or meaningless, I'm likely to construct some new beliefs to accommodate my experience. Imagine, for example, that the book in your hand suddenly felt extraordinary, and that every time the telephone rang, you sensed it was something important, and that the way people blinked their eyes felt like it meant something. As the chain of misperceived insignificance grew, you might start to wonder if you'd been transported to a higher level of consciousness—or perhaps were the victim of a well-organized conspiracy. This is how the delusions (the false beliefs) of psychosis arise."

This might be the first time you've heard marijuana can cause psychosis, possibly because of the confusion around how marijuana is classified pharmacologically. Dr. Christine Miller told me, "A patient doesn't have to exhibit all the symptoms of psychosis to be diagnosed with a psychotic disorder, including schizophrenia. I think psychotogenic is the best term because it implies causation and pertains to all symptoms of psychosis without wading into the complexities of what type of hallucinations and under what circumstances."

Here are the classifications:

1) DEPRESSANT: Slows down brain and nervous system activity. Calms nerves, relaxes muscles, and encourages sleep. *Examples*: Alcohol, Xanax, Valium

2) STIMULANT: Increases brain and nervous system activity. Makes users alert and encourages activity. *Examples*: Caffeine, Nicotine, Adderall, Cocaine

3) HALLUCINOGEN: Interferes with the brain and nervous system and distorts perceptions of reality (visual hallucinations, seeing things that aren't there). *Examples*: LSD, Mushrooms, PCP, DMT *(not marijuana!)*

4) PSYCHOTOGENIC: Induces psychosis, including delusions, delirium, and auditory hallucinations (as opposed to only visual hallucinations). *Examples*: Ketamine, PCP, amphetamine, cocaine, methamphetamine, dextromethorphan (cough suppressant), marijuana[69] (especially—but not only—if exposed during early adolescence)

After Johnny died, I found this email note he sent to a professor at UNC the morning following the 3:00 a.m. incident, "It's concerning a somewhat manic episode I had last night after I finally, finally connected some pieces. Yesterday I broke up with my girlfriend, who I in turn found out was cheating on me with someone who called himself my best friend. I'm just emotionally damaged and cut off a lot of fake a$$ people yesterday, but that was literally it. I know there's been a lot of drama caused by it, and I see now I could have handled the situation better."

His IdRaHaJe friend later told me that before Johnny's psychotic episode, he didn't think marijuana was causing his mental health problems. He said the mental hospital doctor had misdiagnosed him with THC abuse. After the episode, however, she said he made the connection. They drove with some friends to pick up dinner, and he told them all of the cars were chameleons and not actually cars. She asked him if he knew how crazy that sounded. He said, "I need to get rid of the marijuana but just can't do it. Would you help me get rid of my stash?" She agreed to help.

When they got back to school, they drove his car to find a dumpster. She described the contents of his large handbag full of marijuana flower, dabs, oil, pipes, a pen, and glass products. With her encouragement, he tossed it all in the dumpster and told her, "That felt so good. That's a good step." She admitted she *did* report Johnny had expressed suicidal thoughts. But instead of putting him on an M1 Hold, the university officials just moved his dorm room. I'm still angry about their decision to this day.

His IdRaHaJe friend described Johnny as a kind, loyal, generous, and great friend. She was very upset by his passing, and it's been comforting for both of us to talk.

I could also see the psychosis in his writing. In his school papers, I found this YouTube video script he wrote a couple days after his mental break:

> Well, first things first. I am truly, genuinely sorry to all those I have affected with my reckless actions, and the interference my childlike wonder with which I view the world has caused on people's lives, either directly or indirectly. And that's just the truth of it. I am a child, and I always will be easily distracted by many games, and that is never a bad attribute to have. The children of this world are the future, and I fundamentally believe they need to be nurtured in a world that produces safety and allows them to explore the world around them, in REAL life, not behind a full screen. In a sense, it can definitely be okay to view the world behind a screen whatever that means to you, but at some point, every one of us will have to make that decision to move out of our mom's basement. Don't get caught up in the past, don't let it slow your roll or divert your gaze from YOUR truth, the meaning you find in the little things that happen in the world around you and define where you look to the future. Whether you move from your parents early on or collapse with them when they eventually leave, the sad truth

of life is that there's so many of us now, we couldn't possibly know where to stand. And you and anyone else can never be told where to stand, because directing someone in that way causes friction, which can break the big picture. I've learned recently it is okay to live your life undeclared, because your truth will come to you. It's patient, like time. Secondly, I am a liar. If we could view this complex pattern of a world without the hundreds of shades of grey that come with it, I think the black and white picture would all have to do with people's true intentions and the reasons WHY they lie, their truths. Third, I AM a joker, for better or for worse. I have all this green poo inside my brain wreaking havoc, that's been there for quite a long time. And no one's been able to tell me what's wrong with me, despite me constantly wanting to find out. I've come to the realization that it isn't entirely my fault. It all has to do with the paradox that the nature vs. nurture argument represents, which basically sums up our life experiences. This is going to be a controversial opinion. Take it with a SINGLE grain of salt, as you should everything else in your life. On the other hand, we also live as a constant reflection of our credit, the values, truths, and beliefs OTHERS put on you, regardless of their validity. As I was telling someone in the library the other day, everyone lives as a constant confliction AND reflection of their experience and credit, until one outweighs the other. Always try to balance both or you WILL drive yourself crazy. But here's the kicker: it's ironic to a certain degree, but neither experience or credit have ANY intrinsic value, and they are always going to change based on who you are, where you are, and when you are. Everyone in this world defines their own self-worth as a battle between the two, but the battle is never ending. So, stop fighting. Drop your ego, and you can let your true self emerge, victorious. Stay salty.

April 20, 2019 — Arrested and Admitted

Johnny started calling me again. He continued making bizarre claims about UNC secretly being an FBI base and accused John and me of "being in on it," but he couldn't say what, exactly, we were in on. "Oh, you know, Mom, don't pretend," he would say. He said he was fine and refused to let us come to see or get him. My only comfort was that he wasn't expressing suicidal thinking to me as he did before.

Two weeks after his mental break, he suddenly decided to drive home in the middle of the night. I have no idea why, as he didn't call us with a heads-up. Perhaps he realized he was sick and not in his right mind. Since he had thrown out all of his marijuana, perhaps he was feeling extreme withdrawal effects. We were asleep, so we didn't even know this was happening. I don't like to think about how fast he must have driven home because his car literally broke down on the highway. He called John to tell him he was stuck on the side of the road. John called AAA and upgraded our plan to have him towed home. The tow truck hauled his car to our house while he rode in the passenger seat. After his death, we saw the Snapchat photos he sent about his car breaking down and riding in the tow truck.

The tow truck arrived, and John had the operator leave Johnny's car parked in front of our house. Johnny came inside, talking a million miles an hour and saying we were "in on it." We tried to talk with him and said, "Son, please relax. We are not 'in' on anything. Please let us help you. You really need some immediate mental health attention. Please come with us to the hospital so we can have you evaluated properly." Johnny refused. He scared us with his behavior, and James was soon awake with all of the commotion. I was concerned Johnny would become violent. We knew we could not allow him to stay in the house in that state and didn't know what to do.

John told him, "Son, you won't be able to sleep in the house in your state of agitation. I don't want to call the police."

Johnny offered, "I'll just sleep in my car." The weather was mild, so we thought that was a decent alternative for the middle of the night, and we'd talk him into going to the hospital in the morning.

In the morning, our next-door neighbor texted me to tell me Johnny was sleeping in his car in front of our house. I texted back and explained he was experiencing mental health issues, and we appreciated them letting us know and would take care of it.

Because he was 18, Johnny had withdrawn his permission for me to get information from his psychiatrist's office; however, we could GIVE information to them. He had stopped seeing the male psychiatrist and was seeing the Psychiatric PA. I would have never allowed this as he needed to be seeing a licensed doctor, but I no longer had a say in the matter. I had been texting information to her about everything he had been saying to me in the previous two weeks. This was the first time he had demonstrated psychosis, but she couldn't intervene because the university was handling it themselves. She was incredulous they didn't refer him to the mental health system or call the police. But knowing Johnny was a good liar, I'm sure he convinced them he was fine. The Psychiatric PA was unable to do anything while he was at the university since Johnny didn't request help.

I immediately texted her to tell her he was in front of the house in his car and asked what to do. She said to call the police, which we did, and we were told there is nothing illegal about being in your car in front of the house. He wasn't a harm to himself or others. I reported back to the Psychiatric PA, and she instructed me to not engage him but to call the police again and have the officers call her. She told them her patient was sleeping in his car in front of our home because he thought the FBI was watching him. She requested they place him on a mental health hold to have him evaluated. That worked.

It was one of the hardest things we've ever had to do—watch out the front window as the police took him away in handcuffs. We didn't tell them to stop because we knew he'd had a psychotic breakdown and needed help. Because of the poor outcome from his stay at Denver Springs, the Psychiatric PA instructed the police to take him to Highlands Behavioral Health System instead, which was also near our home.

This time, instead of being in the depression ward, the doctor admitted him to a wing with people experiencing psychosis and other mental illnesses. The doctor called me about trying to control his psychosis with an antipsychotic, but it was critical for Johnny to stay off the marijuana. His urine screen was positive for marijuana but no other substances. On the "Informed Consent for Psychotropic Medication Treatment" form, he was prescribed an antipsychotic medication called Abilify. Johnny signed his name and agreed to take Abilify on April 22, 2019. We were so relieved and hopeful that with this medication on board, he would come out of the delusion he was experiencing. He just needed time for his brain to heal while off the marijuana.

The next day, we could visit him. Johnny was full of hatred and vitriol toward both me and John, but mostly me. I'd always referred to myself as "his punching bag." I was the person he knew would love him unconditionally, no matter what, and he knew I wouldn't stop loving him if he said horrid things to me. We ate a meal together in the cafeteria, but he was sullen and ignored us. I went into a "sharing session" with him and his social worker, where he proceeded to tell her everything was my fault. He said I was "in on it," and he hated me. I told him he needed to be in a place where he could be helped. He blamed me for what was happening to him, and it broke my heart. All I wanted to do was help him, but in his mental state, he saw it as sabotage.

When Johnny left the room, she assured me it was just the delusion talking and said he didn't know what was real because his mind was playing tricks on him. She encouraged me not to take it personally. Of course, it's hard not to take it personally when your beloved son is calling you names in front of a stranger.

They could only keep Johnny for three days, and he was released under the condition of a Partial Hospitalization Program (PHP) beginning on April 25, 2019. Sure enough, he checked himself out of the program. Then she said that, unfortunately, she did not see a path for him to come home because it wouldn't be safe for him to be around me alone in that state. She told me about a center for young people ages 15 to 24 called Urban Peak. She had called to confirm they had a spot for him.

Urban Peak is a wonderful non-profit organization in Denver that provides services for young people at imminent risk of becoming homeless. They help youth overcome real life challenges and become self-sufficient adults. The people there required Johnny to be sober and said they would help him find work and affordable housing. As much as we hated him not being with us, we knew he would need a new start once again since he would have to disenroll from his second university. So, we agreed to allow him to be discharged there.

She also suggested we get him into DBT therapy. When I asked what that was, she explained, "There is evidence that Dialectical Behavior Therapy (DBT) helps change behavioral patterns such as substance abuse." I promised I would investigate it, and they listed it on Johnny's continuing care plans, along with medication management.

April 25, 2019 — Urban Peak

Today, Johnny wrote the following in his journal, "Mom is pulling strings in Highlands Ranch. Has my psychiatrist working against me. Need to change all my numbers, need to change everything associated with them, need to lawyer up. STOP getting caught in Catch 22s, stop overthinking, and stop underthinking. Everyone knows what's going on with me at any given moment. Need to change what I can, step by step. My future name, Jonnie — lead by example. Change bank statements, make online presence, new psychiatrist, primary care physician, go to library to change passwords, sell stuff on Craigslist."

Johnny stayed at Urban Peak for a couple weeks. The people were a wonderful help during this difficult time in his life. In fact, at his memorial service, we asked for donations in Johnny's name to be directed there (this was before we created our own 501(c)(3), Johnny's Ambassadors). We were thrilled that more than $5,000 was given to Urban Peak in honor of Johnny. We need more programs like it to help youth who are unable to be at home with employment and housing. So many people see youth living on the street and wonder, "Where are their parents?" Hopefully, now you know, and you'll see places like this as a huge blessing to those needing help.

Sadly, two weeks after he started taking the Abilify, Johnny broke out in a rash or hives all over his body! This was potentially a life-threatening allergy, so he had to discontinue the medication immediately. It had been starting to help, so this was a real setback and a deep disappointment. (The more frequently a mentally ill person is switched from medication to medication, the harder it is to assess the effectiveness and ensure compliance.) He was instructed to make an appointment with his psychiatrist's office for follow-up on April 29, 2019.

Johnny no longer had a car since a mechanic confirmed his transmission was shot. So instead, we planned for him to take the light rail since there was a stop close to Urban Peak. We would then pick him up at Lincoln Station RTD station near our home. (This was where Johnny would later jump to his death.) We planned to have lunch, shop for necessities, and then take him to his appointment at the psychiatrist's office that afternoon.

While waiting at the light rail station, unknown to us, Johnny met a woman (an angel). I learned about her on International Survivors of Suicide Day, ONE YEAR after Johnny passed, and it was a difficult weekend for us. A stranger named Jill Parry wrote to me out of the blue. She had read a story about Johnny written by the Epoch Times[70] and couldn't believe it. She had met Johnny in April 2019 on the light rail and took a selfie! (By the way, in the story, Johnny says he's homeless, but he was living at Urban Peak.)

Here is her story:

In April of 2019, I had the opportunity to travel to Denver with my husband on a business trip. We stayed in a hotel in Lone Tree, Colorado, and during the week, I tried to busy myself while my husband worked. I would walk to the closest shopping area while enjoying the crisp, dry air and abundant sunshine. What surprised me was how unfriendly people were. Often while walking, people would turn away instead of returning a friendly smile and simply did not want to engage.

After a few days, I became increasingly lonely. By Thursday, I called our son during his lunch break to check on our dog and chickens but really wanted someone to talk to during my daily walk to Target. I asked him to pray for me and my unusual feelings of loneliness, as I'd never really experienced that before.

That night when my husband got back from the jobsite, he persuaded me to take the light rail into downtown Denver the next day. One of my biggest fears is of the unknown, and I hesitate to do something I've never done before that moved me out of my comfort zone.

The next day, on Friday, I decided to make the trek to Union Station in downtown Denver by myself! I didn't know the first thing about purchasing a ticket and navigating the light rail. A sweet elderly man must have seen my confusion and helped me out. I sat on the bench waiting for my ride and that's when God sent me a new friend.

Before I left our hotel room that morning, the Holy Spirit told me to put a ziplock bag into my purse because I would need it. I always travel with ziplock bags because they're handy for so many things. I know better than not to obey the small voice and tucked the bag in my purse.

So, I'm waiting for the light rail train to arrive, and a young man sat on the ground next to the empty seat beside me. I told him I wouldn't bite and invited him to sit on the bench next to me. He laughed and took me up on my offer. I asked him his name, and he replied, "Johnny."

I asked him if he lived in Lone Tree, and he said he was from Highlands Ranch. I shared with him that riding the rail was a new experience for me, and he assured me it was no big deal. Johnny ended up sitting with me, and we had an amazing conversation. He shared with me that he was homeless (by his own decision) and had an appointment that afternoon with his psychiatrist for some mental illness he was struggling with. He pulled out a list of medications he was supposed to be taking and said he experienced all kinds of side effects and hated them all.

I commented that I thought he might be really good at math, and he said, "Yeah, I scored a perfect score on the SAT in math." Johnny was trying to decide whether he wanted to change the spelling of his name from Johnny to Johnie and asked what I thought. I told him I didn't have an opinion one way or the other. We were so engaged in conversation that Johnny missed his stop. That's when he decided to ride to Union Station with me. I asked him if he was hungry, and he said he was, so I bought him lunch at Anthony's Pizza & Pasta.

Before we started to eat, Johnny looked at me and said, "You're a Christian, aren't you?" I replied, "Yes." He asked if I would like to pray for our meal, and again I replied, "Yes."

He could only finish one slice of pizza as they were huge. He said he would like to take the extra slice with him, and that's when I pulled out the ziplock bag. He said incredulously, "You have a ziplock bag?" I said, "Yep, the Holy Spirit told me I would need it, and I obeyed."

I asked Johnny about his relationship with the Lord, and he said he believed in God but just wasn't sure how He fit into the equation of his life. He told me he was raised in a Christian home and was raised in the church. I told him it was okay to have doubts but that he could only run from God for so long, because He would pursue him, because He loves him so very much.

When we were walking, Johnny said, "You remind me of my mom." I asked him about his mom, and he proudly told me she was a productivity speaker and traveled all over the world. He told me stories of traveling with her a lot when he was younger.

We talked about his family, and Johnny expressed how his younger brother was outgoing and good at everything. I looked at Johnny and said, "So what you're telling me is you don't measure up." He looked at me quizzically and said, "Yeah." I emphatically told him those thoughts were untrue and that God made him unique and special and being an introvert was of great value.

We walked around for another hour, stopped in a candy store off Market Street, and then Johnny needed to make it back to his psychiatry appointment. I asked him if we could take a selfie, and he willingly agreed. Johnny then asked if I wanted his phone number, and I told him I did because I wanted to pray for him and keep in touch.

A couple hours later, Johnny texted me his phone number, and I sent him the selfie we took. I let him know I was praying for him and what an amazing young man he was.

Two months later, I heard from him again. He apologized for not having my number as he had switched phones during that time, but he was back on the other phone. I sent him a link to the Ted Talk by Susan Cain called "The Power of Introverts." After that, we had no more contact.

I was a new subscriber to the Epoch Times newspaper and received the October 14, 2020 edition in the mail. As I walked home from our mailbox, the article about Johnny's death by suicide jumped right off the front page at me. I could barely breathe. Tears were streaming down my face as I tried to tell my husband what was wrong. Words wouldn't come out, and it took me several minutes to pull myself together enough to read the article.

I'd kept the text message exchange and picture of Johnny and me on my phone for a year and a half, reminding me to pray for him. That's when I knew I needed to contact Johnny's mom, Laura, and tell her this story.

There are no coincidences. I believe meeting Johnny was a divine appointment that day in April of 2019. I thank God for the privilege of spending a few hours with this very special young man and the joy he brought to a stranger with his kindness. God has him now.

Love,

Jill Parry

I rejoiced in my son's value of altruism and am comforted by Jill. Even when he was sick, Johnny demonstrated how we can be a blessing to others in time of need.

Because Johnny was VERY late getting to the light rail station (we didn't know why, and he didn't share about meeting Jill— ever), we didn't have time to get lunch or go shopping. We drove straight to the psychiatrist's office to see the Psychiatric PA. She wrote in her notes (which I didn't see until later), "Abnormal thought process, paranoid, persecutory delusions, poor judgment/insight, disorganized thoughts, not where he wants to be in life, paranoid against parents, Urban Peak employees, diagnosis schizophreniform." She prescribed Latuda and gave him several sample packets to get him started while we had the prescription filled.

April 30, 2019 — Back to UNC

Unknown to us, Johnny was still communicating with the student affairs office about continuing his education and moving back to Greeley to find a job there. Obviously, he was smart enough to know the university would be a better situation for him than Urban Peak.

At the same time, we were in contact with the hall director about Johnny's situation. We explained what happened with his mental health (since Johnny had left there suddenly) and that he would be withdrawing from the university. He told us how sorry he was to hear what happened and said it would be okay to drive up that weekend and pick up his things from his dorm room.

After we'd made the 90-minute trek to UNC, we checked in at the front desk to get his keys. The hall director I spoke with originally wasn't there, and a different person was on duty. He said, "I just need to make a phone call to get verification," and went into the back. He came back and said, "I'm so sorry, but I'm not authorized to give you the keys to Johnny's room. The student affairs office has been in touch with Johnny, and he wants to return."

"Return?" I said, "He's struggling with drug addiction and mental illness and has Fs in all his classes!"

"I'm sorry, ma'am. Johnny specifically disallowed you to remove his possessions."

We were so frustrated that the hall director had given us permission, just to be thwarted and blocked by UNC. The situation continued to be ridiculous. We need legislation to allow a parent to help their mentally ill children who pose a danger to themselves and protect them from self-harm until the age of 21.

I unleashed my fury in an email to the student affairs woman. She wrote back, "Laura, I am terribly sorry it was a wasted trip. I apologize if this was my fault. I assumed communication had taken place between the housing department and you. If it didn't, I apologize that the issue of permission was not clarified before you made plans to come up. I am sure this is like the bitter icing on the mental illness cake. I cannot imagine how difficult it is for you to see your bright and wonderful son coping with this terrible illness. I appreciate the boundaries you are setting for yourselves. Would you like me to keep you informed of what is expected of him to be able to return to UNC?" Of course, I said yes.

She further explained that Johnny would need to have approval from a psychiatrist to prove his ability to benefit from higher education. He would also have to be compliant in the recommendations from his discharge and have regular appointments with a psychiatrist. Well, I knew that wasn't going to happen because he had checked himself out of the program he was supposed to be in.

Then Johnny's IdRaHaJe friend found out he was at Urban Peak and somehow arranged a university bus to get him from Urban Peak and take him back to UNC. It was all so convoluted. Suddenly, Johnny wasn't at Urban Peak; he was back in Greeley, living in the non-bugged room. At least, thank God, he was on antipsychotic medication. That would hopefully help him recover his sanity, even if that's all the mental hospital stay did for him.

Then the student affairs woman wrote to me again, "We have allowed him to return to his housing for the short-term while he has left. We will be working with him and his current treatment providers to find appropriate treatment here in Greeley. He has a hold on his account and cannot register until he is compliant with his treatment." So, I sent her his medical records from the psych hospital that he was supposed to be on meds and in an outpatient program.

Meanwhile, the room and board payment we'd made for the semester ran out on May 5, and he had to move out of the dorm. They allowed him to move to another house on campus and rent a room at a weekly rate. Johnny said he was going to stay in Greeley for the summer to work and recover. So, we drove back to UNC again to help him move his possessions from the dorm to the house. He was still talking gibberish, so I was dismayed the medicine wasn't helping him.

Apparently, Johnny was registered for an outpatient program in Greeley starting May 8. He never showed up because he had no intention of being in a program. He simply said whatever he needed to say to get what he wanted at that time.

Johnny used this time to start applying for jobs. He called me, excited to tell me he had landed a job at Panera Bread—in Englewood, not Greeley—right down the street from where our daughter Meagan was living at the time. He said he was starting in ten days.

"Wait, what? I thought you were going to work in Greeley this summer. We just moved you into your new house."

"Nope. I've decided I need to get far away from this s**thole."

I was baffled but then realized he must have refused to comply with the UNC requirement to get the proper mental health care required by the hospital, so maybe they finally did something to help him. But I was also slightly irritated because he would need our help to move *again*. We would need to find something close so he could walk to work.

I made 100 phone calls (okay, not that many, but it felt like it) to find him a place to live within walking distance to his new job. I put an ad on Craigslist and received several responses. The next Saturday, we arranged to meet with the available rentals on the same day, back-to-back. We drove all the way up to Greeley, picked up Johnny, drove all the way to Englewood, looked at houses with rooms for rent, and then drove all the way back to Greeley.

It was exhausting. Two of the places he refused to live in because as he said, "They were talking about me in subliminal messages." One he disqualified when the guy said, "bad luck" twice. One guy was asleep, and we woke him up when we knocked. He came to the door, completely stoned out of his mind. We said, "Goodbye," turned around, and walked away.

We finally found a place where two 24-year-old young men lived—college graduates just getting started on their own. The roommate who gave us a tour of the house was going to work afterward, so he had on a nice shirt and tie. I thought he looked normal enough. The deal was Johnny would get the entire basement to himself, *and* they owned a dog. So, we accepted, and I paid the deposit. Johnny would move in on May 15. Happy and hopeful once again.

May 6, 2019 — Public Outlets

Meanwhile, back at UNC, Johnny had a week left on campus, and he decided he would start a YouTube channel. We only knew about this from the videos we found in the deleted items on his laptop after he died. We tried to find the YouTube channel, but I don't believe he actually posted the videos. The first was titled "YouTube Video 1."

It started with Johnny playing a psycho scream sound he had downloaded. He came on the video and said:

> I'm sorry about that. Genuinely, I am. I know that hurt your ears probably, but I needed to be heard, and I needed to surprise you. I needed to get your attention. So, are you still listening? Good. My name is Johnny Stack, and this is my YouTube channel. If you can't see by now, I am very amateur at this. I'm new to this video editing and shooting, and I'm figuring it out the best way I possibly can as I go along. Mainly, I wanted to say why is this a secret video if it's on

YouTube. Well, I've been in other secret videos in the past, especially that got a lot of hits, but they were never my work. They were never something that I intentionally created. They were a result of carelessness, not creation. It was a result of being in the right place, time, and circumstances. But I'm done with that.

The next video, titled "YouTube video 2," said:

Hi there. My name is Johnny Stack, and officially, my life is a mess. I am very lost, and I don't know what the next step is, but I thought the very next step would be trying to make a video. And it doesn't really matter what that video is. It could be anything. It could be me embracing the meme; it could be me not embracing the meme; it doesn't matter. It just means that I have to get myself out there. I think the very next step is me creating a short story. I've come up with many ideas of how I should have a public outlet of myself, and none of them have really worked. I've had many different ideas, but I think the next step is me actually sitting down and creating the rest of this story and having at least some idea of what the next steps should be. So, I'm thinking that once I finish this story, I may get someone to animate it; I may not get someone to animate it. But that is the very next step, so stay tuned. I should also add this is primarily going to be a gaming channel. Right now, this is going to be a short story based on recent events that have happened to me and what I should do about those events. But I don't really have the resources right now in order to start recording gaming videos; I don't know how to do that with the current resources I have right now. I'm just recording this from a laptop. I don't have a PC setup. I'm broke. I'm trying to figure out housing. Once I figure that out, that will work a lot better for me. I'm going to have to do a lot of grinding to get there. In the meantime, I wanted to at least have public outlet of myself. So, I'm going to publish this video, and it doesn't really matter. As soon as I can actually start building up my fan base and people who really like me, the sooner I can do that the better. I think this is the very next step of creating some outlet of who I am. So, yeah.

May 12, 2019 — Mother's Day Fiasco

I asked Johnny to come home for Mother's Day weekend to be with our family. When he begrudgingly agreed, I felt happy, even though he was still being cold to me. As a surprise, we bought tickets for everyone to see *Wicked* at the Buell Theater in downtown Denver. Meagan, John, and I had seen it three times, but the boys had never seen it. We planned to go to dinner at the Oceanaire restaurant before the musical and enjoy a nice dinner together.

Since Johnny didn't have a car, Meagan picked him up from his house at UNC and brought him back to Highlands Ranch. Heeding the warning from the professionals, since we weren't sure if he was compliant with his meds and was still exhibiting psychosis, we made a room reservation for him at the Marriott down the street, right next to the light rail station. He was pleased to be spending a few nights in a nice hotel "where someone will pick up after me," he said.

While there, he recorded YouTube video #3:

All right, I'm not exactly sure where to start this video, but I'm going to do my best. Recently, I have been branded as a terrorist. And that has been done because of many actions I've done but specifically because of one action. Recently, I was up at college, and for whatever reason, I was going through a manic episode, and that reason was related to the stuff I was doing and who I was dating at the time. I've figured out that she was a complete psychopath since then. But now, I'm pretty screwed because of what I did. And what I did was I used a lot of words such as bug. For example, in elementary school, I used to be really into the science of entomology and bugs. Well, while I was up at college, I kept repeating this over and over and over again. Right after, I had this manic episode and screamed at 3:00 a.m. in the morning which went viral. And at the time, nobody knew everything that was going on, and so a lot of the hype was building up because of that. Since then, I have been exposed. A lot of my actions and things I've done in the past like four years for example have been exposed. And I can't control that. But what I can control is the mistakes I make from here on out. I know that was a mistake, but it was not completely my fault. I did not know what I was doing at the time. It was completely out of impulse. Part of my mental illness—I do have a mental illness—is that often, I have zero filter with what I say. Instead of preparing for moments, I decide to wing them. And also, with that is the complete inability to hold and retain a lot of information—my memory is very bad. What goes with that, my attention span is incredibly hard for me. It's hard to keep focused on one specific thing at a time. I would just take this moment to apologize and say all of those actions and everyone I impacted as a result of my actions, I did not mean to. It was not my fault. It was something that was completely beyond my circumstances. It was my fault, but there were so many other factors in play. I handled those factors completely bad. And also, I would like to take this time to thank the people who have truly believed in me and still do believe in me and have resulted in everything that's been going on. Words are hard for me right now, but I just want to tell you I truly am sorry for the things that I've done. Thank you. I would also like to add, my name is Johnny Stack, and I have been branded as a terrorist, but I am not a terrorist. Everything I did was out of complete stupidity. I hold none of those actions to be intelligent in any way whatsoever. I was viewed as someone who can be learned from, and that was part of what I wanted to do. I want to be viewed as someone who can lead by example instead of by actual knowledge. In this entire situation, I was leading by example, but not because of me, because of you guys. For that reason, I just need to thank you, again, just thank you so much for this entire circumstance that has happened. There is nothing like it that will ever happen to me again. And for that, I thank you so much.

The next morning, we picked Johnny up for our Mother's Day festivities. We brought him home, and John and James were there. He was delighted to see Lily and enjoyed playing with her. We made brunch, and he gave me a Mother's Day card he picked out and paid for himself. It simply said, "Thank you for knowing what is best for me, even when I don't know myself. I love you, Johnny." I was elated. I still have his card. It's one of my most treasured possessions.

When we arrived at the theater complex that afternoon, we parked on the fifth level in the parking garage. Johnny went over to the railing and looked down at all of the people milling about in front of the theater.

"Do you think they would catch me if I fell?"

My heart skipped a beat, "No, I don't think they would see you in time."

He started *really* leaning over the railing and looking down below. And then he turned around, leaned *backward* over the railing, and spread his arms open.

"WHOAAA!" He pretended to fall and watched for my reaction.

I quickly grabbed his sleeve and pulled him back, "That is not funny, Johnny. Please stop it."

Johnny smirked at me and walked toward the elevator. It was very disturbing, and my heart was pounding. (Little did we know at the time that he would later die this way.)

While we tried to enjoy a light conversation at dinner, Johnny sat and stared as if catatonic the entire time. He would stare at one person and then the next. Then he suddenly announced, "I know what you're all doing, and you need to stop it. You're all subliminally talking about me and trying to humiliate me. I know you're all in on it."

"In on what?" James asked.

Johnny snapped, "You know exactly what you're doing. We are all going to sit here in silence. Just stop talking." Wide-eyed, we glanced furtively at each other and finished eating in silence so as not to disturb him.

When we were finished and preparing to leave, Johnny declared he wasn't going to the musical. He very loudly called me a b***h and again repeated we were all talking subliminally about him the entire time. People around us sensed the disturbance and looked over at us. As we exited the restaurant, he started screaming loudly in front of the passersby. I turned and quickly walked down the block toward the theater with Meagan and James while John stayed with Johnny to try and reason with him. We had an understood signal that sometimes I needed to get out of there to keep from upsetting Johnny. We were like oil and water sometimes.

Meagan, James, and I waited on the corner of the next block and could still hear Johnny yelling. After ten minutes, John appeared with a sullen Johnny, and we all walked together to the theater in silence. John calmly said, "Johnny changed his mind, and he is coming with us." (He had no way to get back as he had no money, and we were his transportation.) The musical itself was uneventful, except that Johnny wouldn't let me look at him; however, he seemed to enjoy the performance.

From that dinner forward, we knew we really had to watch what we said around Johnny because the paranoia made him believe everything had meaning. Amazingly, on the way home, there was a ladybug on the windshield. I *completely* forgot I wasn't allowed to say the word "bug" (or "fish" or "luck" either). I absentmindedly commented there was a bug on the windshield, and oh, my goodness! Johnny started a screaming tirade in the confines of the car.

"You are so stupid! You need to watch what you say because people are listening to our conversations. You can't say the word 'bug' because *they* hear us through our phones. Yours is listening to you right now."

Then, he continued speaking into the air to no one in particular, "I am giving my confession to the government agencies. I did it. I take full responsibility for lying about the bug."

Then he announced to us, "I'm quite famous because the Patriot Act is in place partially because of me. Millions of people know about UNC Greeley because I went there. UNC owes me hundreds of thousands of dollars for making them famous."

I noticed he had tape over the camera on his phone. (At one point, he had six different devices, including burner phones he bought that he believed couldn't be traced.) When we got home, he would not log in to our home Wi-Fi network without using a private VPN he bought and insisted we change the password on our network. We had bought him the iPhone the previous year, but he asked for a different phone since his was bugged. So, I gave him my previous Samsung Galaxy phone, and he spent the evening setting it up and complaining about how awful it was. "Hey, at least it's not as bad as the iPhone for tracking purposes," he informed me.

Johnny had an appointment with the Psychiatric PA the next day, so he spent the night again at the Marriott. I emailed her that evening and told her all about the Mother's Day fiasco. She emailed back and said his meds clearly weren't working, and he needed to be on something stronger. The next day, she changed his meds again to one called Vraylar. I was worried because that was the third antipsychotic in the last few weeks. It just seemed like she was guessing. She gave him a few samples, and we picked up his prescription before driving him back to UNC.

"We'll see you in a few days to move you to your new house," we cheerily told him. John and I drove home in silence, absorbed in our worry.

CHAPTER 6:

THE RISE
AND FALL

May 15, 2019 — New House—Again

The big day arrived when Johnny would be starting his new job. We drove up to UNC one *final* time (and we haven't been back since), retrieved his items, and drove him to his new house in Englewood. It was a nice setup with good Wi-Fi, a big sectional couch in the living room area of his own basement, and a big television. The dog was friendly and took a liking to Johnny right away. We made a trip to Target to get some new items, including a bathroom shower curtain, throw rugs, and food, to hold him over until he could start earning money and replenishing his checking account.

Right before I went to bed that evening about 11:00 p.m., I received a text from Johnny's new roommate.

"What is wrong with Johnny?"

"What do you mean, exactly?"

"Johnny told us the FBI is after him because he's a terrorist."

"What happened that triggered this?"

"We had a little beer and smoked a little weed. I offered him some, and he took it."

"Oh, my goodness! He is in recovery from marijuana and hasn't had any in six weeks. Do NOT give him any, ever again!"

"You should have told me."

"Johnny is nineteen and a young man. He needs to learn to handle his own affairs without his mother violating his privacy. That isn't something you need to know to rent him a room. He should have told you himself he can't have marijuana and refused it. We will not speak of this conversation to Johnny."

I hung up the phone and ranted to John, "Seriously? One time he's offered weed, and he accepts! When is he going to learn his lesson?"

I talked to Johnny the following morning, but I didn't throw his roommate under the bus. He said he hated his new roommates because they were "mean to him," which let me know they wouldn't give him any more weed. He said he was used to living alone in a private dorm room, and he did not like having roommates. I groaned inside, knowing this was probably code for needing to move him again.

He called me later that day. He sounded a bit panicked and on the verge of tears.

"Mom, I can't find my meds."

"Which meds? The Vraylar we just picked up a few days ago?"

"No, my desvenlafaxine. I can't find it."

"Johnny, I filled a ninety-day supply and brought it to you at your house at UNC. You should have over sixty days left."

"I know! I remember having it. I remember seeing it in my desk drawer at UNC. Now I can't find it."

I drove over and helped him look through everything again. Indeed, it was just gone. He claimed someone at UNC stole it, but why would anyone want to take something that doesn't make you high? And he could lock his bedroom door. He only had a few days left on the prescription, so I called the psychiatrist's office, and the Psychiatric PA called the insurance company. Cigna wouldn't cover lost medications, so they refused to give him another 60 days. Then she called in Cymbalta and explained how to divide the rest of the tablets so he could gradually switch over to it. It didn't work as well.

After a couple weeks, Johnny's job at Panera seemed to be going just fine. He was getting up, walking to work, doing a good job, and receiving a paycheck. But then on Monday, May 20, he had a full-on panic attack. He called me and expressed what sounded like suicidal thoughts.

"Mom, I just don't know if I can do this."

"Johnny, I'll be right there."

We were supposed to go to James' Senior Honors Night that evening but explained to him we needed to pick up Johnny and calm him down. James smiled bravely and said he understood—he was used to taking a back seat to his older brother. I texted the Psychiatric PA and told her what was happening. She said he was likely experiencing side effects from switching anti-anxiety meds. She suggested 100% CBD oil (from hemp with no THC) might calm him down.

So, in the middle of a late-season snowstorm, we drove to Englewood to get Johnny. I hugged him and told him it was going to be okay. We got into the car and started driving. I turned to talk to him in the back seat.

"Johnny, what do you want right now in your life?"

"I don't want to live here anymore. I don't like working at Panera, and I don't like my roommates or living in the basement" (as I suspected).

"Okay, sweetie, let's make a new plan. Why don't you go back to school again in the fall? You can take a single class at a local community college such as Arapahoe Community College or Colorado Technical University. That way, you can make new friends and get back into your computer and math. You'll be a part-time student, so we will supplement your housing costs. You'll still need to work, so you can pay for some of your living expenses and take care of yourself. We'll help you look for a new job down closer to Highlands Ranch. You can move into our condo, so you'll live closer to us."

"Wow, that sounds really nice. But I thought you had someone in the condo?"

"We do," John said. "But we'll give him thirty days to move out, and you can move in on July 1. Mom and I have already discussed it. So, keep working your job at Panera, and we'll put the wheels in motion, if you agree."

Johnny seemed relieved and said that sounded like a good plan.

"Meanwhile, you're probably having a reaction from switching meds, so why don't we try some CBD oil drops with no THC?"

Johnny couldn't believe we were uttering those words, but he perked right up. So in the middle of a huge snowstorm, we found ourselves driving to a dispensary for the first time ever. John went in alone. (This wasn't a medical dispensary, or Johnny would have been able to go in.) John sent us photos of CBD oils with no THC. Johnny picked a purple one, and John bought it. That seemed to make Johnny happy as he read the instructions and tried a drop under his tongue. I thought it was all hokey, but hey, the Psychiatric PA suggested it. We crept back to Englewood at 25 miles an hour in the snowstorm. *I'll be glad to stop driving all over creation once Johnny moves into our condo,* I thought.

By mid-June, Johnny seemed to stabilize. I told the Psychiatric PA I'd seen a shift in behavior and language and asked if it could be the CBD. "No," she said, "the Vraylar is working." Oh, right! It had been nearly a month since the Mother's Day fiasco, and he wasn't making delusional statements any longer. Or when he did say them, he seemed to challenge himself that it wasn't correct thinking. He went for his regular appointment with her. She texted me afterward, indicating he was doing better and the delusion seemed to be under control. She warned me it could be six-to-twelve months before he could be weaned off the antipsychotic to see what kind (if any) of permanent damage had been done to his mind from the marijuana. Above all else, *he must stay sober off the marijuana.*

There was one big problem. Johnny and the Bad-News Girlfriend (BNG)—the one who had slapped him in the face and received a year of diversion for domestic violence—had somehow found each other again. From what I can tell from their texts, he contacted her. She was still dabbing daily and struggling with mental illness. My suspicions were confirmed when she picked him up from his house in Englewood and brought him to our house. There she stood in our kitchen. *Oh no*, I thought, *this is not going to be good.*

We had called Johnny because we had a surprise for him. One of my dear friends, Tessa, got a new car, and her loyal old Prius was sitting out on the street. She knew Johnny's car had broken down, so she gave him her Prius. It just needed a new battery, and it was good to go. When they came into the house, I told him the good news, and he was jubilant! He jumped up and down like a little boy, so I jumped up and down with him. He hugged me, thanked me, and hugged me again. BNG just stood there and stared at him. I was worried again.

I told him, "Don't thank me; thank Tessa!"

"I will," he said. "I will go over there and thank her and Charlie." Tessa later told me it was a conversation she and Charlie will never forget. Johnny was genuinely grateful and humbled by their generosity.

July 1, 2019 — The Condo

We reminded Johnny of his commitment to be sober from marijuana and drugs. In fact, we made sobriety and medication adherence conditions of moving into our condo. We decided, given the alternative, we would allow him to use his Juul vape in the condo because he was still hooked on nicotine.

Here is the new "lease" we signed which was really a revised behavioral contract.

Johnny agrees he will:

1) Work 30 hours minimum each week.

2) Attend school part-time (one class to start) while living in the condo. If Johnny fails or quits school, Johnny agrees to move out or pay full market rent. This is the third attempt to pay for school, so any future schooling will be reimbursed upon successful completion only.

3) Pay $800 a month to cover rent and inclusive condo expenses. The difference will be considered room and board for school.

4) Continue to take Vraylar and Cymbalta or other medications as prescribed.

5) Abide by a ZERO TOLERANCE policy for marijuana, alcohol, or other drug use of any kind, except medical prescriptions and CBD oil purchased by Mom and Dad. Eviction proceedings will follow immediately if this condition is violated.

6) Meet with a psychotherapist, therapist, or group at least once a month.

7) Respect our property — no destruction. Respect us — no emotional or verbal abuse, name calling, screaming, or swearing.

Mom and Dad will:

1) Forego $1700 a month in rental income and allow Johnny to live in the condo.

2) Pay for all condo expenses outside of the $800 a month, including utilities, phone, television, and Wi-Fi.

3) Provide an allowance for food, gas, and necessities.

4) Provide insurance, car maintenance, school expenses, and medical needs.

With excitement all around, we moved him out of the Englewood house and into our condo. We used the Nextdoor app and found items he didn't have, such as a king-size bed he wanted for the large bedroom. A kind friend of Tessa's gave him a practically new IKEA couch, and other kind people donated end and coffee tables. He had a nice set-up when it was all over—one that any 19-year-old young man would be thankful to have, and Johnny was grateful.

Now that he had a car, he continued to drive 30 minutes each way to work at Panera while he looked for a job closer to us. He wanted to go back to work with animals again. He really enjoyed the condo but commented how quiet it was when he got home. He said his former friends no longer wanted to associate with him because of the bad choices he had made, and he expressed regret for some of his decisions, such as selling marijuana.

He was seeing BNG a bit, but he still seemed a bit down without anyone else to talk to. He called me one day and said, "I'm really sad about everything today. Just as my life is getting better, I'm realizing I don't have the ability to go back and make different choices. I'm stuck with the results of the decisions I made, and all I can do is move forward."

I encouraged this line of thinking and tried to give him pep talks. We talked about what he could do to find new social interests. He expressed an interest in writing poetry and told me about "poetry slam" events where poets could share their work with others. He said he would start working on a new poem and got excited about that.

We would have him over for dinner quite frequently because he didn't have any interest in learning how to cook and was tired of microwave food and pizza. He knew from living on his own previously how hard fast food was on his budget. We talked a lot about his sobriety and marijuana. (I didn't know it then, but I later read a text string between him and BNG on July 31, and he took a dab with her.) The notes from his July 31, 2019, appointment with the Psychiatric PA say, "Wants to reduce dosage of Vraylar next month (twitching). He states, 'Surviving is a noble fight.'" In the box marked "Status", she checked, "Better."

August 1, 2019 —
Happy Days with Billy and Beagles

These were happy times, finally. A month after he moved into the condo, he seemed to be almost normal. We were cautiously optimistic because I knew BNG was dabbing, and Johnny might not be strong enough to resist, despite his best intentions. He was stable on his medications, not saying bizarre things, sober (as far he told us), living in our condo, enrolling in a new school, driving a new car (for him), and working for pay. He could have been just fine.

(I hope by reading Johnny's story this far, you can see that Johnny recovered from a suicide attempt and a mental breakdown once the marijuana was discontinued. It IS possible for your child to recover, so don't give up and don't despair. Keep trying!)

As mentioned earlier, Johnny (and I) loved the singer Billy Joel. For Johnny's 16th birthday, we had decided I would take him to NYC to see Billy Joel at Madison Square Garden, but Billy had to have sinus surgery and rescheduled the tour. Then we had to cancel the second attempt in October 2017 when Johnny ran away from home. We finally got to see Billy when he came to Denver in August 2019. I bought Johnny tickets right up front. Johnny and I sang every song together, and I finally thought I might have my son back. I was hopeful for the first time in a long time.

Johnny had a great voice. He leaned over and told me, "Third time's a charm, right, Mom?"

"Your patience has won out, son!" I replied.

I have beautiful memories of him smiling and happy that night. Our good friend Andy Lawrence also purchased seats for John and Meagan as a gift. We met up at the intermission and bought Johnny a Billy Joel shirt which became one of his favorites after that. I included it in the quilt I had made from Johnny's t-shirts after his death.

The next happy thing was a puppy! I had read a story about a man with a German Shepherd puppy who said his dog was the only thing that kept him from killing himself. At 50 pounds, our dog Lily was too big to live in the condo complex, which limited dogs to 35 pounds. So, I raised the question to John about getting Johnny an emotional support puppy. I believed it would help Johnny not feel so lonely when he arrived home to an empty condo. In addition, with something else to take care of other than himself, it might make him more responsible. John was against it at first since we didn't allow dogs in the condo previously, and he was afraid it would ruin the carpet. Eventually, he came to see that it could be a good idea. (I can be quite persuasive!)

We didn't know how a puppy could work practically. Johnny was working evening shifts at Panera from 4:00 to 10:30 p.m. Then, he'd stay up late watching television and playing video games, so he would sleep until three in the afternoon. I couldn't imagine that schedule and lifestyle would allow him to take care of a puppy.

I talked with the Psychiatric PA about a dog for Johnny, and she thought it was a great idea for him. She wrote a letter for him, saying, "Johnny has a documented mental health disorder per DSM-5 criteria requiring an emotional support animal to maintain functioning in the community." I talked with Meagan about the possibility of getting him a puppy. Our dog Lily is a one-family, only-pet dog, and she wouldn't take kindly to another dog if Johnny proved to not be responsible enough. Meagan loved the idea for him and wanted a dog herself, so she said she would take the dog if Johnny couldn't take care of it.

With great fanfare, we announced to Johnny that we planned to buy him a puppy so he would have something to come home to. He jumped up and down with excitement, just like he did when he got the car. But first, we told him, he would need a job close to home so he could come home on his break and let the puppy out. He would need to get morning shifts because the puppy wasn't going to be able to wait that long.

Right away, Johnny started looking for a new job. He called PetSmart which was literally three minutes from his condo. Yes, they were looking for a kennel assistant, and he had experience from his prior vet job. The next day, he went for his interview and was hired. He would start August 22. He was over the moon!

So, we started looking at puppies. At first, we considered French Bulldogs because he said that's what he wanted. There were a lot of Frenchies available. Who knew there could be so many Frenchie breeders in one city?

On August 12, 2019, Johnny called me from Just Pets, a pet store near us. "Oh, Mom, there is the cutest little beagle puppy here," he said. My heart melted. When I was a small girl, our family had a beagle named Bingo. I had shown Johnny a photo of me as a baby with my mom holding me on Bingo's back like I was riding him like a horse. My sister-in-law Melanie also had a beagle named Scout. He *really* wanted that puppy, so we gave in and bought it for him. Johnny named him Benji.

August 16, 2019 — University #3

Johnny had a new puppy, and his new job was beginning soon. He was also starting college again at university #3, Colorado Technical University. For the first time in a long while, life was grand. His first class was a required introductory class called, "UNIV104: Academic and Career Success." The first assignment was to complete a "Discussion Document" about himself. I'm still struck by the difference in his writing when he was sober and recovered versus using and psychotic.

Here is Johnny's paper:

Hello, everyone! My name is Johnny Stack, and I'm from Highlands Ranch, Colorado. It's a place that's commonly and fondly referred to as 'The Bubble,' because everything there seems to reflect a status of perfection and cleanliness. It is the epitome of suburbia; kempt and large houses, always-mowed lawns due to the homeowner association's strict regulations, and fancy sports cars everywhere you go. It's a very high paying area in terms of careers and the cost of living there and boasts a low crime rate. The crime rate is so low it sometimes seems as if the police's only job is to pull over teenagers, give out MIPs, or give out tickets for tinted windows. All in all, it's quite a unique place to have grown up. The following are my answers to several questions regarding what college and college success mean to me.

1) Why are you in college? Primarily, I decided to apply for college because I want there to be some significant meaning in my life later. Not to say that you can't have meaning in your life without college, but for me, I feel like college opens doors to new opportunities and through it, I'll accomplish much more in my life. Utilizing my strengths, I hope to finally find my purpose in this world and my passion using what I've learned in college.

2) What experiences have you had that might help prepare you for college success? To be quite frank, I've really had next to NO experience outside of high school that might help me prepare for college success. However, although I haven't quite fully experienced it yet, I know college is a completely different ballgame. Throughout high school, I was diligent with my academic life. I always turned in assignments on time, showed up to class, and achieved a 4.0 every year except for my senior year. Some of my experiences in High School may have inadvertently helped me prepare for

college through the few examples where I was independently learning and showed determination through struggling through obstacles and concepts that I couldn't quite figure out right away. Those notions that I couldn't quite understand or get a grasp of took a lot of persistence to understand and problem solve for. For example, in a lot of my honors and AP classes, a lot of the knowledge we had to figure out on our own. Specifically, I can remember my Honors Biotechnology class and taking a little bit more than a month to complete a project where several classmates and I had to design and create an article about a topic of our choice. It stretched my skills in doing independent research and because the project entailed working with classmates, that has also helped prepare me for situations in college where I must utilize the help of my peers and be a team player in order to succeed. I feel that through that conglomeration of ideas and projects throughout High School that I had to persevere through and show grit, they have helped me become a better candidate for college success.

3) What does success look and feel like to you? To me, success means truly learning something and getting the most out of the experiences we have in this short life and contributing something unique and meaningful for the betterment of mankind and humanity. In other words, I think success means truly making a positive difference in the world. I understand I don't have to be the next Bill Gates or Mother Teresa to cause an impact, however large or small, that could benefit at least one other person. To me, success looks like doing something, whatever it may be, in order to cause a lasting change that can help somebody or multiple people in some way. To me, success feels like making a difference using my experiences here and elsewhere to feel needed, to feel like I truly belong somewhere, and I have a reason for existing.

4) What goals have you set to achieve success in your life? Primarily, my number one goal in life right now I've set over the years and have just now set in motion, is to obtain a degree in computer science or computer information science. I aim to acquire this degree so that one day I may join a software or game design company or corporation that emulates and reflects my own personal values, who finds use in the skills that I am still developing currently and will continue to develop, so that I can feel like I'm needed and have feelings of belonging at that institution. Now, that is the overall, long-term goal, but that doesn't mean I haven't set milestone goals to achieve what I need to in the meantime, until that glorious day comes. One of those was completing high school, and beyond that, learning to live independently. I graduated from high school last year and immediately moved out of my parents' house, firm in my resolve to live independently. It's been a bit of a struggle this past year financially and in other ways, but I am positive that my decision to leave the house I grew up in will set me up for the future better as I'm more acclimated to adult living sooner. As I've learned, adulting is hard.

This paper was interesting to read after he died because he said, "I haven't quite fully experienced it yet" with regard to college, and he "graduated from high school last year." However, he doesn't mention the two universities he attended in between. He also fibbed a bit, saying he graduated high school and then "immediately moved out" of our house. In fact, he had moved out many months prior. I don't think his writing was delusional as much as he didn't want people to think any less of him and wanted to present himself in the best light. The part that said, "To me, success looks like doing something, whatever it may be, in order to cause a lasting change that can help somebody or multiple people in some way" made me proud. He really did believe that, and I try to emulate that in my own life.

His next assignment—to write about the values he thought were the most important in life—was August 20, 2019:

Values I Believe are the Most Important
by Johnny Stack on 8/20/19

1) Altruism — To me, altruism means being selfless or giving to other people, even when there may be nothing to gain and something to lose. Altruistic people do things for the collective interest instead of their own. Practicing altruism is important because it helps benefit the whole of society and mankind. Also, being giving to other people will help yourself in the end, because altruism promotes a brighter future for everyone. Helping other people helps yourself, and it just feels good. As the saying goes, what goes around, comes around. Some argue that altruism is naturally encoded in our genetics because it helps keep our species alive when we cooperate. There are many ways that we can practice altruism, and though it should maybe be practiced more, it occurs all the time. From volunteering at your local homeless shelter or soup kitchen to even simple things like giving presents to the people close to you, putting a smile on someone else's face and giving back means the world, regardless of how big the selfless act is. For example, I practice this day-to-day in often not-too-impactful of ways, such as letting someone go ahead of me in traffic, giving money to homeless people and people who I see are desperate, giving my spot to someone on the light rail if it's pretty packed and they could use the seat more.

2) Patience — In my own words, I would say patience means being able to wait, even in stressful and infuriating situations, often to achieve a better result. Patience is a very important virtue to practice, because if you expect immediate gratification from most things, often you will leave disappointed. Many good things take time to blossom to reach their full potential, and there is no use in getting frustrated. While facing difficult or challenging situations, it's always best to just take a few deep breaths and de-stress yourself, so that you can proceed with the clearest mind to make the best decision. Other coping exercises such as taking a break from what's causing you stress or doing something you love can help de-escalate your emotions in intense scenarios. I practice patience every day by doing a myriad of things, such as when the person in front of me on the highway is going ten under, or when there's a line at the grocery store, or when my mother has stretched out a phone call to 25 minutes.

3) Conviction — I think conviction means showing confidence in what you believe in and know is the truth, and to stand by it. Though it may appear to be cliché and overdone, the biggest role model in my own life is my mother, Laura Stack. She is one of the most dedicated people I know to her profession, which is being an author and a speaker. She travels across the world, speaking about time productivity and using her books as references. She truly is the definition of a competent, assured professional and she always believes in what she's doing. Her leadership skills that she's developed throughout her life have led her to where she is today and creating her own independently run business, The Productivity Pro, and being a symbol of conviction to me and many others.

4) Enthusiasm — Enthusiasm is approaching every obstacle or situation with the utmost of optimism and cheerfulness. Enthusiasm is essential to practice, because if you enter a situation where you're thinking negatively, the outcome will also most likely be negative. We literally are our headspaces, and emit different energies based on our moods and perspectives. These energies are contagious, and how you behave could potentially impact someone else around you. If you go into an event optimistically and thinking positively, regardless if you logically think the opposite. You're more likely to accomplish what you desire and succeed more when you are in control of your own attitude. We can practice this by finding the good things in even dire circumstances, because there is always a silver lining to every misfortune. This is practiced every day personally by reminding myself that sometimes wonderful things can come out of meager situations, doing my best to have a smile on my face, and thinking positively even when it's not the easiest thing to do.

5) Gratitude — Simply put, expressing gratitude is showing you're thankful for what you have, or a kind act. Most people practice gratitude at one point or another, but I believe it's crucial, because so often, we take what we have for granted. For example, there is no other you in this entire universe. The chances of you being born are 1 in (let's just say, a lot), and that is incredible in itself, and worthy of appreciation by every single person. If you're able to appreciate what you have, you're also able to succumb to the dreaded realization that there are MANY people out there who have it a lot worse than you do. We can practice this by knowing that even though you may not be the most privileged person in certain regards, we should be thankful for every little thing that we do

have. I practice this by always showing my appreciation to those who support me, including my friends, family, and coworkers, and by being thankful that I have all the necessities — a roof over my head, food, water, a bed, and much more.

His next assignment was due on August 27, 2019. Apparently, the assignment was to write a gratitude list for five days. Here's what we found on his computer:

Johnny Stack
UNIV104 Gratitude Journal
Due: 8/27/19

8/24:
Pool next to where I live
Gym next to where I live
Laundry machines in my place
Family
Society

8/23:
Brushing my teeth
Shelter
Have enough to afford food
Using my brain; retention and memory
Clothes to wear

8/22:
First day of work, went well
Sunshine
Had fun playing video games
My phone
Running water

8/21:
Sleeping in my bed
Balcony I can chill on
Listening to music
Enjoying showers
Driving my car

8/20:
Was able to present without too many nerves, much better than
I used to be.
Got an A on my presentation.
Made it home safe from class.
My puppy went on his puppy pad like he's supposed to instead of
the floor.
Having a class to go to in the first place, being able to go to
college.

At the bottom of his log was a summary paragraph called "The
Expression of Gratitude":

> Overall, I think this exercise that was assigned to us for the
> purpose of making us think about, be conscious of, and
> appreciate the little things that we often take for granted,
> was entirely enlightening for me. There were so many ideas
> I had for things I was grateful for on a daily basis, more
> than just the ones I wrote down, and I think that actually
> taking the time to reflect on things that might otherwise not
> be noticed, just goes to show how many things we have to
> be grateful for that we should be mindful of. Often, my life
> cruises by without thinking or acknowledging the things that
> I find joy in or assign significance to, or even less, the things
> I would typically define as necessities. Nevertheless, I have
> found gratitude to be an extremely important value to me,
> especially in my recent years, and even was one of my core

values that I shared with the class in my values presentation. I mentioned in my slideshow an encounter that I had about a year ago with a homeless man named Troy that helped shape me and really assigned, emphasized, and prioritized gratitude as one of my core qualities. To summarize, Troy was a dirty, jobless, homeless man that I had coincidentally met outside of voodoo donuts. He was shoeless when I first walked up to him, but after listening to his story of going from living a fulfilling life with a steady job and a wife to losing everything one day suddenly, he inspired me to start showing gratitude for everything, and to give him the shoes off of my feet as a gift for sharing with me this valuable lesson, which I internalized. The lesson is: It doesn't have to be the grandiose things of life and our material possessions that we should show the most gratitude for. Regarding the most basic of things which many of us own or even simple day to day occurrences, thinking about and expressing gratitude in these situations which we often never even think about is the most rewarding. Overall, this activity has been a great experience and reflecting on it, I think it helped reinforce the notion that I previously had to be grateful for all of the small things in life.

August 29, 2019 —
Old Bad-News Derailer Girlfriend

Anything that makes someone feel the urge to use a drug again is called a trigger because it reminds you of using the drug and getting high. BNG was Johnny's trigger. Reading through her texts with him, she mentioned dabs and wax nearly every day. She was physically and emotionally abusive toward Johnny, and he started smoking again with her. Perhaps if she hadn't come back into his life when he was just trying to go to school again, he might still be alive today. We'll never know. I have forgiven her for her role in Johnny's death because she was mentally ill, and Johnny made his own choices.

One evening, I called Johnny to say hello when I knew he'd be driving to class. He answered and sounded a bit nervous. His tone sounded hollow like he was in a tunnel.

"Hello?"

"Hi, Johnny, just checking in. Are you driving to class?"

"Yeah, yeah, I'm almost there, so I'd better run."

He didn't chat as usual, so that was suspicious as well. I told John about the strange phone conversation, "It sounded like he was in a small space, like a restroom. He said he's on his way to class, but he was nervous and didn't talk to me. I also didn't hear any car noise."

John checked the Sprint family locator app on his phone, and Johnny's phone showed he was still near Highlands Ranch, not near the school. So, we drove over to the condo and used our extra key fob to open the garage. Johnny's car was there in its parking space. We walked to his condo, and when we got to the front door, I phoned him from the hallway before we knocked.

"Hi, Johnny, did you make it to class?" I wanted to give him a chance to come clean.

"Yes, I'm here. I gotta go."

My heart sank. I said, "Then why is your car parked in your garage?"

He was silent, then he asked, "Are you *here*?"

"Yes, we're right outside your door. Will you let us in?" Again, silence.

"No. I'm not feeling well, and I'm angry you're spying on me and don't trust me. Go away."

That's when we knew BNG was there. She had talked him out of going to class, and he was dabbing again. We were disappointed, angry, and worried all at once. (After he died, I went back through his text string with BNG, and on August 1, 10, 13, 23, 29, and 31, they specifically talked about dabbing.)

I instinctively knew that was the end of university #3. We'd gone down this path twice before. We also knew we were confronted with the possibility of needing to evict him from the condo, and that entire scenario exhausted us.

The next day, Johnny called me.

"I'm sorry I lied to you. I just didn't know how to tell you I don't want to go to class. People can be very successful in life without going to college, you know. I'm going to pay you back half the money for the classes I didn't take."

"Johnny, I appreciate the apology, but we need to talk more about this. We're really disappointed about you quitting school again. My guess is you were lying about not feeling well and were using marijuana again."

"You don't know what you're talking about. I'm clean. College just isn't for me."

I should have asked him to take a drug test to prove it, but that wasn't a condition on the lease. That was it. He just quit. We felt like we were holding our breath and suffocating.

So, Johnny wasn't going to college. Our arrangement was if he quit college, he would move out or pay the full rent. We stressed about the thought of putting him out on the street with little money. We worried he'd go back to the bad crowd he had managed to escape and start dealing again. I'm sure we made mistakes in this process, but we didn't know what to do. We decided to allow him to stay there, and we raised his rent $100 to $900. We told him we would start tracking what he owed us, and he could pay us back when he got his feet underneath him. He was so relieved and grateful because he fully expected we'd put him out. We told him we'd figure out the next steps together, but honestly, we didn't know what that looked like.

Over the next few weeks, we didn't see him much as he basically worked, took care of Benji, and spent time with BNG. We knew he was using marijuana again, and we were constantly worried.

September 14, 2019 — To-Do, Bucket, and Life Lists

After Johnny passed, I could access the notes from his phone and see his state of mind. Several people have written to me and said, "Oh, it wasn't the marijuana causing mental illness. Poor thing was depressed." I want everyone to know Johnny wasn't depressed at this time. He had hopes, goals, dreams, and to-do lists. He even wrote in his journal that he was NOT depressed. Here are his notes:

Bucket List

Write a book
Journaling
Go skydiving
Do karaoke in a bar
Fly a kite
Go hammocking
Volunteer work in another country
Help people who need it, give back
Read "what we owe to each other," along with many other philosophical books
Go to the beach with Benji
Go surfing
Japan
Drive a very fast car on the Autobahn in Germany
Have my palm read/future told
Offspring concert
Climb a not easy, 14,000 foot mountain
Hold a monkey
Get my ankle (Achilles heel) tattoo
Work in a haunted house
Ouija board. Do some research first.
Have a completely off the grid, no technology, spiritual journey.
Alaska, Nepal, some shit like that
Be hypnotized
Go on a safari
Go to a club
Fly in a hot air balloon
Fly a plane

Butterfly yoga
Swim with sharks

Life Quotes from Phone
"Who even cares? I do. Because if everything is determined, and we have no free will, then all the stuff we're doing to put more good into the world is pointless."
"I guess all I can do is embrace the pandemonium. Find happiness in the unique insanity of being here, now."

To-Do List
Sunglasses
Deposit checks
Go get BNG Popeyes for lunch
Order BNG candle
Get Borderlands 3
Hang out with Desi today
Conversation with parents
Schedule Benji's neutering
More treats, potty pads
Make grocery list
Clean up/organize condo
Put away laundry

The problem was his continued, high-frequency dabbing which I was unaware of at that time. There are specific references to it in his text string with BNG on September 17, 22, 24, 25, 28, 29, and 30, which tells me that daily dabbing was likely. They started having arguments because she used his wax. He said in one text, "Now I'm out of wax, and it will affect me today thanks to you."

On September 23, 2019, he had an appointment with the Psychiatric PA, and she wrote in her notes, "Stopped taking meds. Parents don't know. Lied to keep apartment. Feels delusions were triggered by triggers (people). Now admits to 'delusions and paranoia' i.e., FBI when hospitalized in the spring; denies suicidal intent." In the box marked "Status," she marked "Worse." She wrote, "Per my observation." Her notes also stated he was "using CBD high-potency smoking (read a study about CBD as a treatment for psychosis)."

CHAPTER 7:

THE DEMISE

October 1, 2019 — Brain Treatment

We needed to try something else. I knew Johnny was dabbing (even before I could read the texts with BNG) because he started the odd talk again. He told me his brain was broken and described it again as "green poo." He said he wanted me to get him a brain scan. I explained, "Sweetie, you can't just go get a brain scan. There must be medical cause, and a doctor must refer you. MRIs and CT scans are quite expensive, so you can't just walk in and ask for one. Maybe we can try neurofeedback or biofeedback. I'll look into some options for you."

Coincidentally, we saw a television commercial that evening for a NeuroStar machine which was advertised as a treatment for mental illness by targeting key areas of the brain. I wondered if it would work for psychosis. I emailed the Psychiatric PA about it and asked whether it would be effective for Johnny. She replied,

"Hi Laura, I think this would be a good treatment option if he is open to it. There are studies showing it is more effective than placebo for treatment-resistant schizophrenia. This would indicate that it would help all types of psychosis type disorders, such as those with just paranoia, as is the case with Johnny."

Since he was so interested in "fixing" his brain, I told him about the NeuroStar machine and the treatment called Transcranial Magnetic Stimulation (TMS). I told him I wasn't sure we could get it approved from insurance as it was very expensive, but we could try.

First, Johnny had to complete an interview with the doctor in the TMS office. After his appointment, the TMS doctor reached out to us and asked to schedule another appointment with the three of us. When we arrived, we all sat down in his office, and he asked Johnny, "Have you talked to them?" Johnny said, "Yeah, they actually already know I'm using marijuana. I've struggled with it for many years as I told you and have been using it for a couple months." The TMS doc said, "To be honest, I'm not sure if marijuana is contraindicated for this treatment; we will have to see what the insurance company says. But you can't use it while going through this treatment, and you must stay stable on the medications you're taking."

Johnny looked at us with those beautiful blue eyes, silently pleading for understanding. We didn't say anything except, "Well, let's pray the insurance folks will put it through."

We completed all the lengthy paperwork and submitted it. Cigna interviewed the TMS doctor and the Psychiatric PA, and the company denied coverage because marijuana was involved. They couldn't be sure the treatment would be effective. Johnny really, really wanted this treatment, and he was so disappointed that we decided to pay for it with cash. Before we could tell Johnny, Cigna notified us out of the blue that they reversed their decision! In fact, we were told the company had no reason to believe the treatment *wouldn't* work with marijuana use, either. This was the first time Cigna had ever done anything helpful. Johnny was thrilled, and we were hopeful once again.

We knew he would try hard to stop the marijuana because the doctor said the treatment wouldn't work if he didn't. We did *not* know at the time that he would also stop his antipsychotic medication. Looking back, I think he thought he should go into the treatment with his brain the way he wanted it *after* the treatment; sadly, he mistakenly thought this treatment would cure his brain. The doctor told him to be *stable* on his meds but didn't say not to *change* his meds before he started. Maybe it was part of his mixed-up thinking. Maybe he thought he was better and no longer needed meds. Medication non-compliance is common with schizophrenia. Patients think they are no longer ill, when in fact, the meds are keeping them from being sick. He needed an antipsychotic on board *more than ever* because of the marijuana use.

I went with him to the first appointment on October 9. (According to his text string with BNG, he had used dabs on October 3, 6, 7, and 8.) During this session, the attendants calibrated the machine. They were targeting a single place in his brain, like a focused MRI, using magnets, so it was completely non-invasive. They set the instrument in a place that made Johnny's fingers twitch involuntarily, so they knew they found the right spot. He was strapped in like a spaceman with a big helmet, and the machine made a loud tapping sound. It made me anxious to watch him, but he was calm and happy. Johnny had to have treatments every day, Monday through Friday and off on Saturdays and Sundays, for 37 treatments *without missing*. Each

Friday, Johnny gave them his work schedule for the following week, and they scheduled his next sessions. We prayed the TMS would be a breakthrough for him. He was so dedicated to attending faithfully—he completed 35 out of 37 treatments without fail. Sometimes he would forget or be late, so the center director developed a relationship with him and would call him to remind him and/or wake him up.

Each session, he was required to fill out a form to indicate his level of suicidality. Every time, even on the day he died, he circled "no thoughts of suicide" and didn't miss a treatment. They sent me a copy of his form, and I saw he had circled "0" on the scale, meaning none. One week before he died, he wrote that the TMS had cured his depression and worked exceedingly well. Sadly, with the marijuana use and no antipsychotic on board, the delusional thinking was seeping back into his mind.

One weekend, James came home to visit from Colorado State University where he was attending his freshman year. Johnny and Meagan both came home to see him. I loved having the five of us at home together again. Johnny was all over the place, jumping excitedly from one subject to the next. He talked about quitting his job. He announced he didn't like the new therapist I found for him, whom he had seen exactly twice. He told us he had an argument with BNG because she went off her meds for her borderline personality disorder and was being difficult. And on and on. Then the delusion from the marijuana use started to rear its ugly head, and I thought the antipsychotic was the only thing keeping it at bay. He said to John at some point in the conversation, ". . . but that's because you're in on it. Actually, I take it back. That's not true. You couldn't be in on it because you would have told me." John and I glanced sideways at each other, wide eyed.

Afterward, I wrote to the Psychiatric PA and told her Johnny had been using marijuana again. I feared the meds or dose weren't working correctly because his paranoid language had returned. The Psychiatric PA said she would tell him to come in for an appointment for a med and TMS review.

The Psychiatric PA confirmed he exhibited disorganized, paranoid thinking after she talked with him. He admitted to her that he had been dabbing with BNG for a couple months but hadn't wanted his mom to know. Then she dropped the bomb—he'd stopped taking his antipsychotic medicine. I felt like I'd been punched in the stomach. She reassured me that Vraylar had a long half-life, so its effects would last for several weeks. Meanwhile, we must do everything in our power to get him to take it again, so I called him.

"Johnny, I'm heading to Target to do some shopping. Do you want me to pick up your refills for you, or do you have it?"

"Mom, I stopped taking the Vraylar."

"Oh, Johnny, why? It was helping you so much. The marijuana will bring back your psychosis, so you really need to keep taking the antipsychotic, or you'll have a breakdown again."

"It's okay because I'm going to be sober during my TMS treatment. The doctor said I couldn't change my meds while I was on my TMS treatment. I hate taking those meds, Mom. They either give me hives, make my face twitch, or make me fall asleep or brain-dead. Besides, you couldn't tell the difference when I'm on it and when I'm not."

"That's not true, honey. I could definitely tell the difference. You really need an antipsychotic on board to control the delusional thinking the marijuana triggers in you."

"Mom, I'm not going to spend the rest of my life taking those medicines."

"We're not talking the rest of your life, Johnny. You know you have to be sober long enough for your brain to heal, and then you can wean off them again."

But there was no reasoning with him. He thought he didn't need them. I braced myself. I didn't know what to do. He wasn't finished with his treatment, and if he didn't finish the course, he couldn't get more in the future. John and I debated pulling him out of the program but didn't, praying to God the treatment would help him. John constantly begged the Lord to heal our son.

October 12, 2019 — The Dab That Broke Him

John took Johnny to see *The Joker* movie, which he loved. He said he related to the Joker's mental illness. Johnny went home and dabbed that evening, as I later read in his text string with BNG. Then late that night (October 13), BNG called our other son, James. BNG told James she was really concerned about Johnny and asked him to please check on him. Startled, James texted Johnny and FaceTimed him. Then James called my cell phone at 2:00 a.m. (What is it about these middle-of-the-night calls?)

"Hi, Mom," James said. "I'm sorry to bother you so late, but BNG just called me and said to check on Johnny. I texted with him at first, and he was acting crazy in his texts, so I called him, and he seemed more normal. But you might want to call and check on him, too."

I called Johnny, my heart pounding. "Hi, Mom," he answered nonchalantly, like he wasn't surprised I was calling that late.

"Johnny, are you okay? James said BNG called and said to check on you."

"Oh, Mom, like I told you the other day, we got into a fight because she stopped taking her meds. I had some choice words for her because she's trying to gaslight me, so I broke up with her."

"What is gaslighting?"

"Mom, that's when you make someone question their own sanity. She's trying to make me think I'm crazy. I'm fine, really. Go back to sleep."

"If you're sure, but I'm happy to come over and talk for a while."

"No, Mom, I have lots to do in the morning, so I am headed to bed." So, I went back to bed—and didn't sleep a wink. I knew he'd had another mental breakdown.

That afternoon, Johnny got into another fight with BNG. Here is their text string I found later:

> Johnny: you called my brother last night
> Send me the screenshots of yalls convo
>
> BNG: i really didnt know what to do. i was expecting you to hate me for getting them involved but i was too scared you would do something that i didnt want to risk it. i thought you were going to hurt yourself
> im really sorry johnny
> i didnt want to call the police because i wasn't sure you were gonna do something and i didnt want them dragging you

off to another hospital where you would hate and blame me.
i just needed someone to make sure you were okay

Johnny: They wouldn't drag me off to a hospital. I would
have just told them the same thing I told James, you're lying
and making shit up
That was none of your business to reach out to him

BNG: i was just worried im sorry

Johnny: My mom called me at 2 am thinking I was gonna
kill my self. Nice.

BNG: i was scared you were gonna johnny im so sorry
i didn't know what to do you called me freaking out and then
blocked me i was scared
Johnny I really am sorry. i know you already said you
believe me, i just really was so fucking scared and i didnt
want to lose you. i know it was shitty to bring them into
it but i was half asleep and i didnt see any other option
and im so sorry. i genuinely just care about you and i want
you to be happy, healthy, and successful. i was very torn
making that decision because i knew it would upset you
but if you had done something to yourself and I didnt do
anything i would have never forgiven myself. i needed to
know you were safe. i love you so much and i care so much
about you. im so sorry youve been thru all this and im
sorry you dont trust me anymore i just had to do the best
i could to make sure you would be okay. i just want you to
be happy

Hours later:

BNG: do you still want to hang out?

Johnny: Yeah, just don't talk about getting back together with me please

BNG: no problem i wasn't planning on it i know you said you didnt want that last night. Rn?

Johnny: No I'm at my parents rn, is 7 ok

BNG: ill find something to do but i do ask please try to like be there at 7, its not a huge deal or anything if i wait i just dont rlly want to but like no rush dont worry abt it

Later that night, around 10:00 p.m., Johnny called me, crying and gasping.

"Johnny, what in the world?! What's wrong?"

"Mom, I'm sitting here in my car, and I'm furious, and I don't know what to do."

"What happened?"

"(BNG) was over at my house, and I asked her to show me her phone, and she wouldn't. She wouldn't leave, so I tossed her phone out into the hallway. She punched me in the face and ran out down the hall. I'm just so mad and don't know what to do, so I'm sitting here."

"Johnny, drive to Skyridge Emergency Room right now and meet me and Dad. I'm calling the police to meet us there. See you in a minute. Go now."

"Okay, see you there."

I called the police and said I wanted to report a domestic abuse incident. The dispatcher said she would have an officer meet us at the hospital.

Johnny, John, and I got to the hospital at the same time. Johnny had a big red cherry mark on his right cheek. I couldn't believe she had punched him again after everything that happened to her after the first time she struck him. I was so proud of him for not hitting her back.

"I'm so sorry this has happened to you, Johnny." He let me hold him while he cried softly. We checked in at the front desk and then sat down. The police officer arrived and took Johnny's statement and photos in an office room in the back.

We went back to his place, and he turned to me, "I'm not going to dab anymore, I swear. This incident with BNG has helped me see, finally, it's the problem. In fact, I'm also going to quit nicotine. I'm going to work on being a better person."

"Love, you know we will help you with all of our power."

"Will you buy me some self-help books?"

The irony of that question made me chuckle.

"Oh my, I have probably 100 of those on my bookshelf from friends—come over tomorrow and take your pick!"

The police went to BNG's house in the middle of the night, arrested her, and took her to jail. Johnny was summoned to court to testify, and they granted him a restraining order instructing BNG not to contact him. After Johnny died, the domestic abuse charges against her were dropped because he wasn't there to testify. However, I was given the opportunity to show up at court for the hearing. By then, the world was dealing with COVID-19, so it was a virtual hearing. I put a photo of Johnny up to the camera, showing his bright-red cheek where she hit him. I told everyone in the virtual courtroom that this woman abused my son last year, she abused him again, and she deserved to be convicted again for domestic abuse. I said I felt sorry for her because of her mental illness, but she contributed to my son's demise by her betrayal and marijuana use. I felt good about showing up for my son and holding her accountable.

Meanwhile, Johnny had started skipping work which I assumed was from sadness, loneliness, marijuana withdrawal syndrome (MWS), and sudden withdrawal of his antipsychotic. He saw the Psychiatric PA on October 16, 2019, after he stopped taking the Vraylar, and she could see the change. In the "Status" box, she checked "Worse," and in the "Judgment/Insight" box, she wrote, "Poor." Her notes said, "Much worse mood/irritation after breakup with girlfriend. Says he's 'not psychotic,' even though he admits to some paranoia. Recognizes he had some paranoia before but now thinks some paranoia is justified (UNC mafia, girlfriend 'gaslighting him,' and mental health providers not caring). Encouraged patient to start the Vraylar again, but he declined. Denies suicidal intent. Educated him about girlfriend's BPD and not to take it personally." She noted a right cheek bruise in her notes (from where BNG hit him). So, without his medication, he was clearly sliding. He first agreed his thoughts were delusional, but at this point, he was saying they weren't.

October 23, 2019 —
Late-Night Condo Visit

After Johnny's death, I had a 90-minute conversation with a good friend of Johnny's, Seneca Rayburn, who gave a eulogy at Johnny's funeral. They met through the National Speakers Association (NSA) where I was president in 2011-2012. Every year, NSA held a youth leadership conference within the main conference. Johnny and Seneca attended it every summer together since they were ten years old, and in 2017, they were leaders together.

Seneca had moved to Colorado to go to college and texted Johnny, asking him when they could get together. In true Johnny style, he said, "I'm not doing anything right now! Come on over," and she did. She stayed at his condo from 10:00 p.m. until 8:00 a.m., literally all night long. They filled each other in on their lives over the previous two years.

Johnny shared with her about his struggles with marijuana. He told her he sincerely didn't want to use it anymore because it had messed up his head. He asked her to help him throw it away to make sure he wouldn't use it. Seneca told me, "He brought the trash can from the kitchen into the bathroom and asked me to toss his stash. I'm not knowledgeable about THC products, but I threw away what looked like sap and some sort of devices to use it. He showed me the CBD distillate that you (his parents) bought for him that didn't have any THC in it. He said smoking CBD distillate would help him get off the marijuana. He told me he stopped taking his antipsychotic meds also because they made him feel terrible. But everything else that night seemed normal."

The next evening, Seneca invited Johnny to come over to her place to introduce him to her friends. She said they were all having a great time playing ping pong. Then suddenly, he seemed to withdraw, and he told her, "I think it's time to leave." He was short with her, as if having a fight with someone. She honestly had no idea what happened and was very confused. She called him later that evening, and he angrily said, "It's so obvious how you were all acting. You didn't really want me there."

Seneca repeatedly asked him, "What did I do?" He would respond, "Stop kidding yourself," or "Stop believing your own lies," and then he told her, "Have a good life." This was the first time Seneca had seen him psychotic. Poor sweet young lady didn't *know* he was psychotic until she talked to me, and I explained that's how the paranoia manifested itself. She was so relieved, I thought she might cry. She had held on to the burden this entire time, thinking she had done something to anger him.

They kind of got it worked out as Johnny did tend to come into his right mind again and realize he'd overreacted. They texted a few times in the days after that, and the last one was on November 18, two days before he died. He asked her if she liked anyone, and she sent him a photo of her new boyfriend. That was the last she heard from him. After he died, Seneca got the cutest tattoo on her arm, just under the bottom line of a short-sleeve shirt. It says, "Hello my friend!" in his actual writing from a note he wrote her in their NSA days.

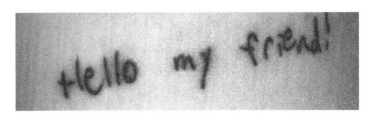

The full sticky note read, "Hello my friend! This year has been so amazing despite you still hanging out with Voldemort, (jk jk♡) but yeah it's been awesome. Your personality is so hilarious and awesome, and I love every minute with you. Plus, our dancing is amazing, I'm going to miss you but I'm glad you're a leader next year :) — Johnny."

Serious about getting off marijuana, Johnny asked us to buy him more CBD isolate to help him stop, which we did. The ingredients didn't list THC, but I was suspicious. I wanted to find someone to test it for me but couldn't find anyone. We did not know Johnny had seen Seneca or that he had tossed his stash.

I found a selfie on Snapchat to an unknown friend dated October 29: "Girlfriend and I broke up, long story, but she punched me in the face, and I now have a restraining order against her. A lot of old friends have changed and extremely dislike me for s**t I did in the past that I can't change, but I'm focusing on becoming a better person right now. Keeping the right influences and connections in my life to becoming who I want to be. I've stopped smoking for almost two weeks now, and I want it to stay that way. My head is already much clearer, and I'm genuinely more happy. I'm being who I am and not worrying about what other people think of me. I don't have anything to prove to people whose main personality trait is smoking a drug."

Johnny really wanted to get better, and I admire him for that. He was talking about his plans and creating new goals to have a new job and a larger place for Benji with a yard by March 2020. This was not the to-do list of a depressed person with no goals (dated November 2, 2019):

To-Do List
Where I can get degree. Do research
Research where to live, where to work
Fundraising to get enough money to move out of Highlands
Ranch and start college
Coursera — check out if accounting is a good fit
Clip Benji's nails
Sell Armani watch — Facebook marketplace
Team trees shirt
Socks from griffins shop
Check out Jiujitsu website
Raking leaves grandma
Clean outside of car
Get oil changed
Write out long-term plan. Strengths/weaknesses, where you want
to be by 21. You need a plot, what you wanna witness with this
life you got
Get more cbd isolate
Start keeping journal/video diary
Volunteer. Trash duty
Check out WallPad
Check out Brilliant.org/WIL
Start philosophy podcast/class?
Learn about the production of music, create an album in the
future
Start studying accounting through an online college

TV Shows to Watch
The first 48
7 deadly sins
Attack on Titan
Fate/stay night

ATLA live action remake NEW ONE OFC
Blue exorcist

Books to Read
Words that work. It's not what you say, it's what people hear
12 rules of life
Self-help leadership
7 Habits of highly effective people
The power of now — Eckhart Tolle

November 13, 2019 — Cannabis Withdrawal Again

At this point, we still didn't *really* understand about today's high-potency marijuana, its addictive potential, and its effects on brain development. Research shows concurrent tobacco use and daily marijuana use makes the withdrawal even worse, and some small studies[71] show venlafaxine can worsen the CWS. This was where Johnny was at this point. The addict basically feels like crap. Until his own dopamine and serotonin neurotransmitters kicked in, Johnny would not feel normal.

We just didn't understand how difficult and critical this phase of marijuana cessation can be. First, we weren't sure he was clean because he'd lied to us for many years about his marijuana use. He'd sworn to John he was clean, and we didn't know this time was different. Second, he had also quit vaping nicotine. He bought nicotine lozenges, so we knew he was having withdrawal effects from that as well. Third, the antipsychotic would have worn off by now, so there was nothing to counter the delusion he certainly experienced. We didn't know how bad it was until we read his journals after he died. He hid it from us. Why he didn't come forward and tell us how much he was struggling, we'll never know. Perhaps he thought he could tough it out. Perhaps he thought the TMS treatments would resolve it, and he just needed to hang in there. Perhaps he was afraid we would take him to a mental hospital again, so he just didn't want to tell us. We will never know. He certainly never mentioned he was feeling suicidal. I guess I thought he would since he had told me the other times. Not *this* time.

November 14-16, 2019 — Johnny's Journals

Journal Entry #1: November 14

Johnny wrote:

> This week has been one of significant internal change, one like I've never had in my whole life. This year has been the most mind blowing, filled with extreme ups, but mostly paralyzing downs. After what happened at UNC, I wasn't sure what to do, but I completely missed my train of popularity and didn't get to ride that wave. It's amazing the way things happened, however, because I wouldn't have gotten the chance to grow and realize what I've realized today if it wasn't for these negative a** learning opportunities. I consistently fell for the bait and bought many people's bullshit and sympathy stories over the past two years, leading myself right into traps, but I didn't care about my own

well-being, so I let it happen. As of today, my depression is almost gone. The TMS has succeeded extraordinarily, beyond what I had hoped. This week I've experienced so much growth, mostly because I trust myself much more now to read in between people's lines and have the realizations that the ripple effect of the whole world knowing about every single aspect of me was never in my head to begin with, but I MUST pretend that it was. All of what happened to me at UNC from January to May was just the plan of what the previous year had been leading up to. I was set up by the mob, again, because I had inadvertently sent some of their members to prison, among other reasons. It started with (name of cheating girlfriend), whose plan to make me a public shit stain psychopath backfired as it spread to beyond way more than just UNC. It soon became the plan of UNC after I screamed at 3:00 AM, started threatening the public safety with my words, and was just a general nuisance, to net this dangerous fish and dangerous because I was clueless and couldn't care what anyone thought about me at the time, out of UNC. I threatened their safety and because UNC was secretly a military base or some type of Federal Institution, one of the core pillars of the United States. This week I learned that NOTHING is pre-determined, and it can be proven that we have free will. I learned this from watching The Good Place, a show all about an interpretation of the afterlife that is very entertaining, thought provoking, and related to many aspects of ethics and philosophy. I just know we have free will; I'm not quite sure how to explain it. "Who even cares? I do. Because if everything is determined, and we have no free will, then all the stuff we're doing to put more good into the world is pointless." More than anything this week, I've learned that all we can do is to live in the moment, in the present. Not to say you should go for immediate comforts like smoking and not do anything responsible. Because what some think is responsibility-lessness bliss is actually an existential catastrophe. The <u>PAST</u> and <u>FUTURE</u> are both concepts; all we have is the current. When everything seems overwhelming, take a deep breath, and focus on the unique insanity of being here now, meditate by blanking your mind and focusing on nothing but your physiological normally automated processes.

Journal Entry #2: November 15 and 16

Johnny wrote:

> Yesterday, November 15 started out on an okay note. From the previous couple days, and me knowing that <u>I had to pretend</u> to be asleep (not knowing the whole world knows about me, which I actually made myself ignore and forget about it because I was so blind to (BNG'S) deception from June 2019-October 2019, because I chose to be convinced by it instead of trusting myself). Well after TMS that day, where (TMS Director) said several keywords and referenced me being greedy in the past with how much I was expecting vs. how much people were willing to give after my loss upon loss upon loss, very much so endless suffering, all of which was self-inflicted, because I didn't know how to cope with my situation in April-May after the 3AM yell at UNC. Well, after (TMS Director) made all these remarks, I took it very personally, especially because the previous day I had messed up with timing, and just being lazy in general after November 13th, when the hype (a little bit at least) came back after I promised I was going to change, knew what was going on, and promised I was going to improve. A lot of people's reactions were, "Well, we'll just have to see about that because you've claimed to know before and broken

about a million other promises, reflected in people like (friend's) snap story. The hype had been steadily building after I dropped some wisdom bombs.

November 17, 2019 — Johnny's Warning

I wrote to the Psychiatric PA, "Johnny is a bit manic. He is running around being super productive. Cleaning, raking leaves, talking a million miles an hour, etc. He says he's quitting smoking, moving condos to save money, getting a new job, and starting school to be an accountant all by March. I am a little overwhelmed by everything he's saying he is going to do and am afraid of the crash."

Earlier that day, John and I had gone to church and had invited Johnny to go with us. That evening, he came over at 5:30 p.m. for dinner.

I greeted him joyfully at the front door, "Johnny!" I hugged him for a long time. I can still remember the feeling of his arms around me and his tight embrace. He was wearing his charcoal gray down jacket. I wasn't expecting what he said next.

"I'd like to go to church now."

I was happy and thought, *Oh, this is fantastic—he wants to go to church! He hasn't been to church in such a long time.*

"Johnny, that was 11:00 this morning. Services are all over for the day."

"I guess it's too late for me."

Did he mean too late to come back to the Lord? "Oh, Johnny, it's never too late. It doesn't matter if church is closed because you don't have to go to church to ask the Lord back into your life. You asked the Lord into your heart when you were baptized at ten years old, and God has never departed from you. Just ask Jesus to forgive your sins, make a commitment to live for him, and ask him to come back into your life."

Johnny was happy with that response and seemed relieved.

We walked to the kitchen and made small talk while John and I finished preparing dinner. Then, standing in the kitchen, Johnny turned to me and pointedly said:

"Mom, I just want you to know you were right. You were right all along. You told me marijuana would hurt my brain. Marijuana has ruined my mind and my life. I'm sorry, and I love you."

He hugged me, and I was so happy he wanted to settle things between us. He could be vicious during his psychotic episodes, and our relationship had been strained for many years. I used to be "his person." I didn't see this act of reconciliation as a suicidal indicator, but it probably was, and I missed it. It makes me sad every time I think about it.

After dinner, he told us he'd finished the original poetry we talked about for the slam contest. I had found a call-in for the "World Poetry Open Mic" at *www.worldpoetryopenmic.net* and sent it to him. He asked if we wanted to hear his poem and visit Benji, so we all went to the condo. For whatever reason, he decided to record himself reading his poetry, a part of which we included in his tribute video.

Here's his poem:

Back Down, To Earth

I'm too impatient, while getting punctured by punctuated punctuality.
The latent world revolves around commas, why you can see the duality.
If they weren't existing, dramas wouldn't give pause while persisting,
That there's no real cause, while wildly untrue, you always say.
Never, have my view, don't sever faith in a conception.
Completely unknown, other than you, stopping, the deception predecessor,
For movement on its own.

Cause commas don't make cents, that's what periods are for.
I wish I could have been less dense and known this before.
So, let's put breaks where they're "supposed" to go, right?
I'd still probably make myself ignore it though. Night.

A new friend named Cynthia McGregory, who also lost her daughter Richelle to suicide, sent me a poem her daughter had written. I told her I didn't understand poetry very well, but Johnny had also written a poem. I asked her if she wanted to read it and interpret it for me. She eagerly agreed, and I sent her Johnny's poem. She said, "Yes, at first reading, it is hard to understand. I think the poem uses punctuation as a metaphor for societal constraints. It is as though, in his psychosis, he has visited another realm, come "back down to Earth" with a sensitivity that has removed the veil of existence, exposing our world in a way that makes it difficult to endure the harsh realities of living, as though even the rules of grammar are part of a larger conspiracy to make him betray himself. Truly epitomizes the existential question for him and Richelle—in the state of mind they were in. I loved the word play on sense and his reference to money in 'cents.' Periods are much more concrete compared to commas, and that's what you need to be to survive in this world. Even though he knows this now, he admits he probably won't listen anyway. He and Richelle would have understood each other very well. Such a tragedy we lost them both. Johnny was fascinating and brilliant. I agree, marijuana for them was deadly…deadly…sigh!"

Wow, I was amazed Cynthia could get all that from his poem! I clearly need to read and study poetry more.

After the poetry reading, I remembered what the Psychiatric PA told me and braced myself to convince him.

"Sweetie, Dad and I see the change in your behavior. I need to ask you to please start taking your Vraylar again. Your desvenlafaxine can't handle the load alone from quitting marijuana as it's not an antipsychotic. You really need an antipsychotic on board to keep your brain from playing tricks on you again while your brain heals. This is really important to me. Please." (We hadn't read his journals at this point and didn't know it was already happening.)

Surprisingly, he agreed, and John and I were elated! We watched Johnny take a pill.

November 18, 2019 — Red Robin

Johnny was supposed to have an appointment with the Psychiatric PA on this day but canceled it. I received a text from him.

"I'm not taking the Vraylar. I wasn't taking it at the beginning of my TMS, and so (TMS Director) says I should not be taking it now under any circumstances. It can mess with my treatment, making it ineffective and causing seizures. I'm not prescribed it anymore because I really don't need to be on it. I had an episode because of nicotine withdrawal."

Then the phone rang. It was Johnny.

"Hi, Mom. How about we all go to Red Robin tonight at 6:00 after my work? I have something I need to talk to you about."

"Sure, Baby, that sounds fun. Everything okay?"

"Yeah, I'll tell you about it then."

At 6:30, John and I were still waiting for him to show up. We'd already ordered his favorite Red Robin Royal burger and Oreo Cookie Magic milkshake for him.

When he finally arrived, he ate a little bit and suddenly announced his news.

"I need to move to California."

"Wait, what? Why? It's November, and there is snow on the ground. I thought you were going to try to move by March?"

"Yeah, I need to get out of Highlands Ranch. I've got to get away from everyone here."

"When do you mean?"

"Tomorrow. I need to pack up and leave. What will I do with my dog?"

"What do you mean? Benji is your dog, so you'll take him with you wherever you go. You'll have to figure out where to work and how to take care of him. Where is this coming from?"

"You are the worst parents in the world!"

Johnny got up and stormed out of the restaurant. John and I looked at each other, mouths open. We hadn't paid yet and didn't know what to do. Johnny had a long day at work, and we figured he needed time to cool off and decompress, so we let him go.

November 19, 2019 — The Day Before

Johnny was off work this day and the next. At 4:21 p.m., he showed up at our house without calling. Our Ring doorbell recorded this entire interaction. He had Benji with him. He rang the bell, and I came out with Lily excitedly running about, jumping up on Johnny and wrestling with Benji. I sat on the porch, and he sat on the porch swing and looked at me.

"I owe you a huge apology. I do not know what I was thinking. I've been an idiot. I really have. And I don't know how to say it other than that."

I should have just wrapped my arms around him and told him it was going to be okay, but I thought about what the Psychiatric PA had told me. Instead, I begged him to take his medication, and we ended up arguing. How we spent our last moments together is my worst regret—discussing medication. I just felt a sense of desperation for him to take it.

"Mom, stop. I'm not going to take that medicine for the rest of my life. It makes me feel stupid, and I'm not going to live my life that way. I love you and need you to promise me that you're going to be okay with me doing it my way."

I didn't know what he meant. Did he mean figuring out his meds on his own?

"Promise me."

"I promise."

John heard this exchange from the front door and came out.

"Son, I don't know what your life looks like without the medicine."

"Well, I do. Anything wrong with my brain I can fix myself. I've had spiritual enlightenment."

"What does that mean?"

He was silent and wouldn't explain. Later, from Johnny's Netflix account, we could see that he watched 37 episodes of *The Good Place* within the last two weeks of his life. We noticed the episodes titled *Pandemonium* and *The Worst Possible Use of Free Will* corresponded to the quotes on his phone. Could he actually have experienced spiritual enlightenment from a fantasy comedy television series? One thing we understand for sure from Johnny's addiction is the power of free will, choice, and independence in destroying your own life. As parents, we should have the ability to take back control of a young adult's decision-making when they are mentally ill. When addicted, they can't see that their free will is causing them to make destructive decisions. The law takes away a parent's power in one day—when the child turns 18, and parents are often powerless to help. We can only watch our children self-destruct.

Johnny didn't verbalize his suicidal thoughts, and we weren't on the lookout for the signs. He had told us—and he meant it—that he would never go back to the mental hospital again.

November 20, 2019 — Death Day

On the actual day he died, Johnny went to his TMS session as usual. Then he got an oil change on his car. He texted John to confirm the type of oil he should put in his Prius. John texted him back with the answer, and then he texted John a copy of his receipt. That was our sole interaction. We know he went to get Krispy Kreme doughnuts, his favorite, because they were sitting on the counter when we arrived, and there was a lone receipt in his wallet.

That evening, John and I were watching television. I was thinking about Johnny and hoping he had a good day off. I was a bit surprised I hadn't heard from him. I remember looking at the clock at 10:15 p.m. before going to bed. I thought about calling him to check in and tell him I love him, but I decided he needed a break from me after the previous three days of emotion. We went to bed.

Meanwhile, around 9:45 p.m., Johnny left his condo. We believe he intended to kill himself because he left the front door of the condo slightly ajar so someone could find Benji, who was locked in his kennel. But there is a bit of a mystery because his house key wasn't on him or recovered by the police. So, there is a possibility he left it ajar so he could get back in. But why he didn't just close it and leave it unlocked steered us more toward the possibility he left with intention.

He got into his car and drove to the RTD Lincoln Station parking garage across the street from his condo. He drove from the first level to the sixth (top) deck of the garage which has no fence except a small rail on concrete barriers that someone can easily climb atop. A fixed video camera films 24/7 and caught the entire incident. We have never viewed nor will we ever view that video because we can't unsee it, and we're certain it would cause trauma. In some ways, we feel blessed we never had to come upon our dead child, as some parents have had to suffer through with a child's suicide. I did, however, request and receive a typed timeline from the coroner's office, so we could piece together the timing of a Snapchat photo he sent.

Here was the chronology:

2155: his car comes up the ramp into the top open-air parking lot
2156: circles the lot
2158: he parks with the front of the car facing the cement barrier
2159: shuts off his car lights
2216: gets out of the car and looks over a ledge and stands on the ledge, jumps down from the ledge and walks around his car and area at a normal pace
2220: gets back into the car
2221: brake lights come on and he backs out
2221: reparks his car parallel to the ledge; driver door is next to barrier
2232:34: he exits the front driver's side door, leaving his door open, jumped up onto the barrier ledge outstretching his arms and pushes off his toes

Between 9:59 and 10:16, there's an 18-minute interval when he was just sitting in his car. During that time, he sent his brother James a Snapchat to tell him he loved him. James replied, "I love you too, Bro." He had seen Meagan recently when he went to see her new house. We saw him the last several days. He went over to Grandma's and raked her leaves for her. We did not see these individual instances as his way of saying goodbye because they all seemed isolated.

Johnny composed his suicide Snapchat note which he sent at exactly 2215 (10:15). It was a picture of his car odometer showing the mileage of 133661. Below the photo, Johnny actually typed out the mileage from the photo and some text. The Snap read, "133661. For every action, there is an equal and opposite reaction. For one extreme to exist, there must be the opposing." James received the Snapchat and just thought it was Johnny being Johnny and didn't think anything of it.

Why did Johnny see meaning in an odd odometer reading? I talked with Dr. Erik Messamore about it afterward. He speculated Johnny saw evenness with the doubling of the number 3, the two 6s in the middle, and the 1s on the end. Johnny thought this was *so important* he needed to post a screen shot so everyone would see it. This way, everyone could see the sign Johnny thought was apparent, and he *was right* about his suspicions. After reading his journals, Dr. Messamore was confident Johnny was experiencing psychosis at the time, due to him perceiving something significant in his odometer reading—an association delusion. In his mind, Johnny was having a tremendous insight he wanted to share with the world. With Johnny getting an oil change earlier that day, Dr. Messamore believed Johnny had no intention of dying earlier in the day, so no one could have seen it coming. Schizophrenics have abnormal impulse control, like a "flare up" of psychosis. Johnny wouldn't have weighed the pros and cons or long-term consequences. He couldn't envision more than one option into the future. Dr. Messamore further told me, "If Johnny were feeling angry or unloved, he wouldn't have died that way. He would have shot himself in front of you or wrote a note that it was your fault. Perhaps he thought he could fly."

I emailed Zerrin Atakan, a consultant psychiatrist at Nightingale Hospital in London and an expert in schizophrenia, to help me understand why this happened. She was kind enough to read his journals and the suicide note, and she gave me this opinion:

> I have read Johnny's notes, he was clearly very unwell and highly distressed as a result of his delusions at the time. I looked at the Facebook you've sent. He was obviously such a lovely person. What a sad loss. I have been interested in the links between cannabis use and severe mental illness (psychosis) since the early '90s following clinical observations when I saw my recovered patients with psychosis becoming unwell again following cannabis use. This led to me wanting to carry out research examining the links. Shortly after, I discovered the difficulties in doing research with an illegal substance, namely cannabis at the time, but persisted regardless, with a group of other likeminded colleagues here in London. After so much research on the topic, I and now many others in the field have no doubt that THC, particularly high dose THC, can trigger an enduring psychotic disorder in those who are genetically vulnerable, particularly if the use is from an early age and is frequent.

Then she was kind enough to schedule a Zoom call with me, and I typed up our call notes. She believed his language evidenced psychosis, specifically persecution delusion. He believed the mob was after him, and he sent some people to prison so some sort of harm was going to come to him. He needed to escape so as not to be captured by his enemies. Her belief was he thought he wouldn't die, as evidenced by him getting his oil changed that day. There was a razor on his bathroom counter, so he shaved because he thought everyone would see him. By jumping from such an extreme height, when he lived, it would somehow show the world he was magical. In his journal, he wrote, "The whole world knows about every single aspect of me." So, he believed he was a very important person and omnipotent since everyone was aware of him. When he said he had experienced "spiritual enlightenment" the day before, she was further convinced he didn't believe he would die. In addition, the video of him jumping off the building showed him spreading his arms out and jumping off his toes, as if he believed he could fly. Zerrin believed he was having a psychotic episode when he left his apartment, and the 3s and the 6s on his car odometer reading 133661 were a "sign" to him that he should do it. He may have heard voices commanding him to do it. In the end, he was clearly unwell because of schizophrenia. However, he was so intelligent, he had moments of lucidity when he knew his brain had been affected by the cannabis. In his mind, this was the only cure.

Added to his marijuana abuse, psychosis, and impulsiveness, Johnny was socially isolated, even though he wanted to live alone. He had suffered the recent abuse and betrayal from BNG. He had a negative attitude toward medication and wasn't following his treatment plan. He referred to his brain as "green poo" and knew something was wrong with his mind, as he'd told us in the kitchen days before. From some of our conversations, I know Johnny had realized how serious his condition was. He used to have a good life and recognized how much he'd lost.

An article in WebMD[72] discusses schizophrenia and suicide, stating, "Schizophrenia is strongly linked to a higher-than-normal chance of suicide and suicide attempts. Suicide prevention can be hard to do, because people with schizophrenia can sometimes act on suicidal thoughts impulsively and without warning." It goes on to say, "The classic person with schizophrenia who attempts suicide may:

* Be a male under age 30

* Have a higher IQ

* Have been a high achiever as a teen and young adult

* Be painfully aware of schizophrenia's effect on them"

November 21, 2019 —
The Call in the Night

Here, I pick up where I left off in the Introduction.

John and I began living every parent's nightmare. While I sat wailing, sobbing into John's chest, he held me tight and tried to talk to the police officer and the coroner. He explained about Johnny's marijuana use and mental illness. He surmised it must have been impulsive, and I still agree with him to this day, because he'd just had his oil changed that day and attended his TMS session as usual. (We later requested a copy of the form he filled out that day at TMS, and he circled "0" on the suicidality question.)

The coroner handed me a clear plastic bag with an orange "Biohazard" symbol on the front. In it were Johnny's items:

- His black NEFF beanie that still smells like the vape he used

- A multi-colored SMOK vaping device

- His Ray-Ban sunglass case with his favorite black with gold frame Aviator Ray-Bans inside

- A Key Lime Chapstick

- His black leather bi-fold wallet which contained a $20 bill, a receipt for Krispy Kreme, his Social Security card, driver's license, AAA membership card, Cigna insurance card, ADP pay debit card, bank debit card, and KickBack points card

Mercifully, the police officer did not tow Johnny's car but left it there atop the parking garage. He quietly handed John the key and softly said, "We left it there for you to pick up."

Two people showed up in our living room, apparently community grief volunteers. They hung back, and the officer asked us if we would like to speak to someone about this. We thanked them but said not right now. It was a nice gesture for two people to come out in the middle of the night to offer support, but a couple weeks later would have been better timing. We never did find out who they were because they didn't leave their cards.

Then the officer said we must decide right then, after we just received the news of our son's death, if we wanted to donate his body. Obviously, time was of the essence to receive his gifts. John and I looked at each other, and although we'd never discussed it with Johnny, we immediately knew this would have been what he wanted. He was to be cremated anyway. We had purchased a double niche at Cherry Hills Community Church Memorial Gardens where his grandfather, John Stack, was also laid to rest. As he wrote in his school paper, his #1 value was altruism, and he spent his life trying to help other people, so we agreed.

The Donor Alliance called immediately. John answered their questions and granted permission to use anything available. In his death, Johnny created a living legacy of generosity with his ultimate gift of love—himself. His gifts included skin grafts, tendons and ligaments, corneas, and bones. They were unable to use his organs due to the manner of his death.

After the coroner and police had finished their reports and paperwork, they told us how sorry they were one final time, and they departed. John and I stared at each other, fell into each other's arms, and held each other, wailing.

I wonder if he left a suicide note? I thought and said, "John, we need to go to the condo, get Benji, and pick up the car." Still crying, we drove to his condo. His front door was slightly ajar. We immediately agreed he left his condo with the intention to die. We went in and closed the door behind us.

Benji was so happy to see us. We took him out to potty and gave him food, water, and love. *He left Benji,* I thought to myself. *This wasn't supposed to happen.* I couldn't imagine the fear and pain Johnny must have felt to be able to do that. I had such compassion for him then.

Just so you don't worry, our daughter Meagan adopted Benji, and he's happy and healthy. My daughter is now married, so today, Benji has a new buddy, Tucker, her husband's Labrador. Benji's doing well in his new life, and we still love it when our granddog comes to visit. Meagan posted on her Instagram, "Few things in life brought Johnny more joy than his pup. Benji reminds me of the best of Johnny. It's the greatest gift, honor, and privilege to adopt Benji and give him all the love Johnny would have given him. Rest easy bro; I'm taking good care of your baby down here."

We frantically searched around for a note. We saw his black-and-white composition notebook—the one he'd just read his poem from only days before—right on the top of the counter where he knew we would find it. We checked the trash and all over the apartment, but that was the only thing he left for us to read. Crying, we flipped open the notebook and found the two last journal entries you read a few pages earlier. We could read how delusional his thinking was about the mob being after him again. Without the antipsychotic on board plus the marijuana use, his psychosis was back with a roar.

On the counter, we saw the box of Krispy Kreme doughnuts (his favorite treat we used to buy him for good grades). Next to it was the dab pen from the Nectar Collector kit, a butane torch, a foul-smelling liquid from where he cleaned the pen's water chamber, and the CBD isolate we'd purchased for him. He must have been dabbing the CBD right before he left the apartment.

We have often wondered if the CBD isolate had any connection to his sudden impulse to die, but the package said it had 0% THC in it. Perhaps Johnny had read something about CBD helping with psychotic symptoms or regulating THC in cannabis. CBD has been used as add-on therapy with standard antipsychotic drugs,[73] but it's not good enough to be a standalone antipsychotic. However, it was a case of "you don't know what you don't know" because we found out the package insert of the FDA-approved form of Epidiolex, which contains CBD, lists depression and *suicidal ideation* as possible adverse reactions. Could this be possible when smoking CBD isolate as well? In the largest placebo-controlled clinical trial[74] among 27,863 patients treated with Epidiolex and 16,029 patients treated with placebo, the risk of suicidal ideations increased one in every 530 patients, and four suicides occurred in the Epidiolex-treated group versus none in the placebo group.

In his bedroom, some of his clothing was still on the ground from after he took it off. It smelled like him. His bed wasn't made. A full prescription of unused Vraylar was on his dresser next to a bottle of desvenlafaxine with the lid off and nicotine lozenges. In his bathroom, his razor and shaving cream were on the counter; he'd clearly just used them. The counter still had water on it.

We gathered Benji's things and went back to our car to retrieve his car. We drove to the garage and sobbed as we climbed up the parking ramp, knowing our son had just done the same thing hours earlier. We got to the top, and there was Johnny's car, parked alongside the cement wall near the far railing. We parked, got out, and looked down. There, we saw the cement curb and paved walkway below which was the last thing he saw before he jumped. John got into Johnny's car, and we drove both cars home.

Unquestionably, this memory is very painful to recall. For many months afterward, I had PTSD symptoms every time I thought about driving up to the top of the parking deck the night he died. I had recurring nightmares, picturing him standing on the cement wall with his arms outstretched. I would wake up in a cold sweat and felt as if I'd cried out in my sleep. Some nights, after not being able to get out of bed from crying all day, I was so deeply depressed that I didn't know if I could make it another night. Sometimes, I asked God why He didn't take me instead. My doctor gave me a prescription that would force me to sleep for a couple months afterward. John and the children, my family, friends, Lily, and the Lord got me through those dark times.

CHAPTER 8:

THE AFTERMATH

November 21, 2019 — The Morning After

We knew it would be a long, horrible day, so we tried to sleep for a few more hours. After a bit of fitful sleep, we woke up and were immediately hit by reality—our son was dead. It wasn't just a dream; we had woken up to a nightmare. We immediately started wailing and screaming, holding each other, not knowing what to do. We knew we needed to call Meagan and James, so we did that first. You can imagine their reactions; suffice it to say it was awful. Meagan came to the house shortly after our call, and James began the 90-minute drive from CSU.

Meanwhile, John wanted to see Johnny. He just couldn't accept that Johnny was gone until he saw him with his own two eyes. He called the coroner's office and insisted we see his body. The coroner said they didn't have a viewing area, so we couldn't come to their office. We were told to call the funeral home. Angry, John told the coroner that unless we got to see Johnny, they could forget about the organ donations. He instructed them not to complete an autopsy until we could identify him.

We called Mike Hefflebower. He had helped us when Dad passed away, and we had identified him the night before as our funeral director. We tearfully explained what was happening and begged him to please go get Johnny from the coroner's office. He dropped everything, picked up Johnny, and brought him to the funeral home. Because time was of the essence with Johnny's bodily gifts (they must be retrieved within 24 hours of death), a loving family kindly postponed their son's memorial service for an hour so we could see Johnny.

Our family arrived at the Hefflebower funeral home about 11:00 a.m. As we walked in the front door, Mike quietly said, "He's in there," and motioned to a room. "Stay as long as you'd like."

We walked into the room, and there was Johnny. He looked like he was sleeping. I ran over to him, shrieking, "Johnny! Johnny!" I lay down on his chest and held him. I stroked his beautiful, soft brown hair that he'd just had cut a few days before. It was short over his ears like I liked and had a wave in front. I stroked his hair over and over and cried all over his face. His face was clean shaven, smooth, and cold (41 degrees, Mike told me later). Just cold, not freezing and not sweating. I heard my wails arise from my mouth as if from another world. I sensed my family around me, crying, and hesitantly touching him. I smelled his clothes. (I still have the clothes he was wearing in a bag to keep his scent.) I beseeched him, "Johnny, why did you quit? Why did you give up? Why did you have to do this to yourself?"

My family encircled me, hugging and stroking me, and we all cried. I inspected every part of him. It was so strange—there was no blood anywhere. He looked so peaceful and beautiful. The lines in the corners of his eyes had relaxed. I touched the mole on his cheek and the scar above his eyebrow from falling at daycare when he was two. I once again thought he needed a facial to get rid of those blackheads on his nose. His fingers were curled and frozen in place from rigor mortis. His knuckles were scraped and scabbed as if they had hit the ground with great force to catch himself. The black body bag was zipped open to his waist. I had an impulse to unzip it and check his legs to make sure he was okay, but I didn't. I held on to him for about 30 minutes and couldn't let him go.

Finally, I went and sat down so others in the family could say goodbye to him. John touched his chest and cried. I took a deeply touching photo of John standing above him. Then I took photos of my dead son, knowing this would be the last time I'd see him. Meagan didn't want to touch him, so John held her while she cried. James stood solemnly, softly crying as he touched Johnny for the last time and said goodbye to his only brother.

I went back to hold Johnny for the last time, softly weeping. Finally, John gently pulled me up and said it was time to leave. The other family, the funeral director, the coroner, the Donor Alliance, and the eye bank were all waiting on us. They had all followed through on their promises.

It came time to say our final goodbyes. I leaned over, laid on his chest, kissed his cheek, and stroked his hair one last time. I looked at him and whispered softly, "I love you, Johnny. I'm so sorry I failed you. I will see you in heaven." I let go, looked at him one last time, turned, and walked away. *Goodbye, my poor, precious son.*

Several weeks later, we received the results from Johnny's toxicology test. The report said he had *no* THC or other substances in his system when he died, just desvenlafaxine (which he went on after his first suicide attempt) and nicotine (from the lozenges). He had told John the truth—he was clean for the five weeks prior to his death. In the end, he made a valiant attempt to be sober and wanted to be a better person (in his words). Johnny dreamed of taking his puppy to the beach and having a career in computer programming. He wasn't depressed, neglected, on drugs, or unloved. He was psychotic, paranoid, and delusional from the marijuana. His torment caused him to take his own life to escape his pain and his imagined persecutors.

We didn't put all the pieces together until after his death when we had better information and access to his devices and journals. When I read his texts, one of the saddest discoveries was seeing he tried to reach out to the TMS doctor on Monday, two days before he died. However, he texted an office number. He also texted the new therapist I found for him (at his request) on Monday, but it was her day off. He texted a childhood friend and didn't get an answer right away. He was crying out for help, and no one helped him, not even us because he didn't text me this time. When I saw these texts, I wept and wept for my poor boy.

I had periods of anger—angry at the marijuana. Angry at the attorneys, lobbyists, and legislators who helped legalize it in Colorado so my boy could access it. Angry at myself for not moving to Idaho or somewhere else where it was still illegal. Angry at the owners and manufacturers of this poison. Angry at Johnny for using it. Johnny's decision to use marijuana led to addiction and psychosis, but it shouldn't have been as readily available as it was. In the end, the blame for Johnny's death lies squarely on marijuana; without it, Johnny would still be here today.

I have stopped blaming myself. We weren't perfect parents, but John and I did the best we could with what we knew. Sleep and a mother's love can never cure the exhaustion Johnny felt. The coroner said that when he did it, he was feeling better enough to take his life because he got some energy back. He survived as long as he did because of who we were as his parents and our love for him. When we looked down deep, we realized his death wasn't our fault, even though it often felt that way.

Johnny simply wouldn't accept our help. He kept checking himself out of every program. He fought my help by withdrawing permission for his psychiatrist, school, and doctors to talk to me. He stopped taking the antipsychotic meds he needed, and his psychosis returned. It was simply too much to quit marijuana, stop meds, quit nicotine, have a new brain treatment, go through withdrawal, and manage the return of the psychosis—all at the same time. There were too many factors against him. It's a tribute to Johnny's integrity that he had apparently recognized the potentially damaging effects of high-potency cannabis use. At the end, he had taken real steps toward abstinence and recovery, but it was too late. The bottom line is a person must want to get better and help himself/herself.

When someone has repeated cannabis-induced psychosis (CIP) incidents, eventually, the psychosis doesn't go away. Johnny was diagnosed with schizoaffective disorder, and after six months, the psychiatrist officially diagnosed him with schizophrenia. The Psychiatric PA emailed me and said, "I don't think Johnny was bipolar, but rather a more pure psychosis like schizophrenia. But he may have thought he was having a bipolar manic episode since those can look very similar to straight psychosis."

John and I couldn't watch our son 24/7, so his time on this earth was limited. We couldn't protect him from himself. Johnny's written journal entries made it clear that his brain had turned on him, and he was not himself. And now, we are not ourselves.

We grieve Johnny's choices but feel relieved he is free from his torment and in the presence of God!

November 22, 2019 — The Next Few Days

The next few days were a blur as we notified family and close friends. I rarely stopped crying, and my head and heart were in constant pain. The Donor Alliance and eye bank were able to obtain Johnny's gifts. The coroner's office did an autopsy on Johnny's body and shared with us that he died within seconds. He would have felt no pain. His cremation was performed two days after his death. I had an overwhelming urge to hold him one more time but knew it was impossible. We asked the funeral director to set aside some ashes which our family members have in necklaces and boxes. He also put some ashes in a portable tube to scatter in Hawaii the next time we visit. I keep a little blue heart-shaped box printed with, "We love you, Johnny," on my nightstand with some of his ashes. Every night, I touch it and think of him. Sometimes, I pick it up and shake it, and I can hear little pieces rattling inside. It's the last piece of him I have to hold on to in addition to my locket of a mother and child that also contains his ashes. I thought about tattooing his name on my Achilles like he wanted to do, which would be fairly appropriate.

Fortunately, it was fall break at CSU because the Thanksgiving holiday was the following week, so James could be home with us during this time. Once James and Meagan announced their brother's death on social media, we also shared the tragic news on Facebook. We'd never experienced such an outpouring of love like we did after the news of his death went public. We received hundreds of cards and gifts as well as a month of meals, organized by our dear friend Ruby Newell-Legner. Never underestimate what a blessing a meal is to a grieving family; it was literally too much to think about eating.

Our pastor, Mark Shupe, ministered to us for hours and talked us through the inurnment and memorial services to come. Donna Carlin, from the church, handled all of the details of the service. John's sister Melanie flew in from Kentucky. Our close friends Mark and Darla Sanborn invited us to their home for Thanksgiving so we didn't have to face the holiday in our home without Johnny.

Two days after his death, some of James' and Meagan's friends helped us go to Johnny's apartment and clean it out. We bagged up Johnny's clothes and personal items so I could go through them at home. We gave away furniture and extra kitchen items to Goodwill. We knew we couldn't just leave everything there, or we wouldn't be able to face our grief head on. We brought home his personal items and put them in his old bedroom for safekeeping. I sent his favorite t-shirts to a company called Project Repat (*projectrepat.com*).

November 25, 2019 — Inurnment

Someone emailed me a beautiful poem written by Anne Lindgren Davison called "When God Comforted Me." I loved it and reached out to Anne directly in the hope of receiving her permission to use it at Johnny's inurnment and memorial service. I wrote, "Hi, Anne, my 19-year-old son died by suicide last week, and I think your poem perfectly reflects the way he felt when he did it—FREE. He struggled with mental illness and addiction issues, and we are only comforted knowing he is with the Lord. I think this poem will bless those who are at the funeral. Thank you for making your poem available."

She kindly responded, "Dear Laura, thank you so very much for responding to my web page. I am very touched that my poem found its way to you and brought comfort as you go through this difficult time. My heart is heavy with your story and your loss. I feel so honored that you will share it at your son's funeral. Please know that you are in my prayers. Most sincerely, Anne Lindgren Davison."

Johnny was inurned with a small group of family and close friends in attendance. A winter storm was due to hit, so it was freezing cold and windy. We bundled up in our winter gear, and our pastor, Mark Shupe, gave a touching message of comfort. I read Anne's poem with John's firm hand on my back steadying me.

WHEN GOD COMFORTED ME
by Anne Lindgren Davison. Used with permission.

Don't grieve for me, for now I'm free,
I'm following the path God laid for me.
I took his hand when I heard him call,
I turned my back and left it all.

I could not stay another day,
To laugh, to love, to work, or play.
Tasks left undone must stay that way,
I've found my peace at the close of day.

If my parting has left a void,
Then fill it with remembered joy.
A friendship shared, a laugh, a kiss,
Ah yes, these are things I know you'll miss.

Be not burdened with times of sorrow,
I wish for you the sunshine of tomorrow.
My life's been full; I've savored much,
Good friends, good times, a loved one's touch.

If my time seemed all too brief,
Don't lengthen it now with undue grief.
Lift up your heart and rejoice with me!
God wanted me now. He set me free.

Reading that was all I could manage. Torrents of smothering sobs wracked my body as John, James, Meagan, and I took turns screwing in the nameplate on the niche. The word "STACK" had been etched into the metal with "John Drew" on the top and "Johnny Kenneth" on the bottom (he never used his legal name of John). If you're ever in Highlands Ranch, Colorado, please feel free to visit Johnny's niche in the upper left corner of the Lily 1 wall in the Cherry Hills Community Church Memorial Gardens, just south of the large Jim Dixon chapel with the steeple and stained-glass windows.

With all our hearts, we absolutely believe God is in control. He certainly knew He would be receiving Johnny into his loving arms. In early January 2020, John and I were blessed to see musician TobyMac in concert in Denver. His 21-year-old son, Alex, had died just a few weeks before Johnny did. Toby sang his newest hit, "21 Years," which beautifully expresses the searing pain and agony of his loss:

Did he see you from a long way off
Running to him with a Father's heart
Did you wrap him up inside your arms
And let him know, that he's home

…

Well until this show is over
And you run into my arms
God has you in heaven
But I have you in my heart

I pictured my own prodigal son arriving in heaven. I thought of the Father running to greet him and receiving him with open arms, and it gave me great comfort.

TobyMac reminded us that because of our faith, we have hope we will see our loved ones again in heaven. TobyMac told the crowd, "God gave us His first-born son, Jesus, so that I can see my first-born son again!" I need to remember this powerful truth again and again as I move through this tragedy.

Johnny, I've loved you for your whole life, and I'll miss you for the rest of mine.

December 9, 2019 —
The Memorial Service

The day finally came to celebrate Johnny's life. I was a nervous wreck just thinking about the major meltdown I was about to have. The night before, my dear friend Stephen Tweed (and his wife Elizabeth Jeffries in spirit) arranged a dinner for the out-of-town guests at a nearby restaurant.

That morning, in addition to our family and friends, Johnny's friends, former teachers, and PetSmart co-workers came to pay their final respects. James' and Meagan's friends attended to support them. My local colleagues from the National Speakers Association and seven fellow past presidents flew in to show their solidarity. In total, over 300 people gathered at the Jim Dixon chapel. (Luckily, this was before COVID shut everything down because the place was packed to the gills.) We were overwhelmed with the incredible expression of love and support.

John, James, and Meagan gave eulogies (the ones you read in Chapter 1), as well as Johnny's childhood friend from down the street, Frank Jose, plus Seneca Rayburn. I was the last speaker and cried through this eulogy for my son:

"These have been the saddest days of my life, so it's going to be difficult to share with you, but the fact that you are all here makes it less difficult. I'm going to cry and may not get through this quickly, but since you are our loved ones, I know you will understand. Even though I'm a speaker, I wrote out every word I wanted to say, so I wouldn't forget anything.

I doubt any of you *don't* know, for reasons we'll never fully understand, Johnny took his own life on November 20, 2019. Johnny had struggled with marijuana addiction and the resulting anxiety and depression and then later psychotic episodes and treatment-resistant schizophrenia. He was admitted to multiple hospitals and treatment programs, saw many doctors, and tried different medications and even innovative brain treatments. In the end, despite our best efforts, we couldn't get in front of the runaway train of mental illness and addiction.

We purposefully didn't hide the fact that Johnny died by suicide because there are more families struggling with mental health issues than we know. It seems that everyone we talk to has a story about drug addiction, mental illness, or suicide in the family. The prevalence among young adults is on the rise, so it's important to talk about it and bring attention to the issue.

As tragic as Johnny's suicide is, the *more* important thing is the life he lived before he made that decision. The *facts* of his life are less important than the *story* of his life—everything that came in between is what's important. I recognize that many of you here never met Johnny, and you know him a bit better after hearing from our family and his friends. You now know that Johnny loved the ocean, amusement parks, and animals. He had a spirit of service, a beautiful smile, and a kind heart.

As his mother, I think the best way I can tell you about who Johnny was is to share from his own words. Three months ago, Johnny enrolled in his third university, Colorado Technical University, where he wrote a paper titled, "Values I Believe Are the Most Important." I'd like to briefly share his five values and tell you a little story about how he exemplified each value and what we can learn from him. On your way out, please pick up a copy of his paper in his own words.

1) Altruism — Johnny said, "Practicing altruism is important because it helps benefit the whole of society and mankind. Also, being giving to other people will also help yourself in the end, because altruism promotes a brighter future for everyone. Helping other people helps yourself, and it just feels good." He really believed and acted on this value. Once he literally took the shoes off his feet and gave them to a barefoot homeless man. He volunteered at church; we

taught Sunday school for preschoolers as a family for several years. He loved being a youth leader at the National Speakers Association annual conventions, giving back to a program he had gained so much from when he was younger. When Johnny was about 15, we were driving north on University a few blocks from here, and it was pouring rain. My wipers were going like crazy, and we stopped at a red light. A man was standing on the corner with one of those SALE signs for a local business, getting absolutely soaked. Without hesitation, Johnny reached down and grabbed my umbrella, rolled down the window and handed it to the guy. The light turned green, and I drove off. I blinked and looked at him and said, "Well, be prepared to be wet," and he said, "Well, he needed it more than we do." I looked back in my rearview mirror and saw the guy, now with the umbrella in one hand and the sign in the other, and knew Johnny was right. In death, Johnny has given life to others. His legacy will live on through the nearly two dozen people who will receive his bodily donations.

2) Patience — Admittedly, it was initially difficult for me to understand how patience could be Johnny's second value because he could be very impatient at times. On one of our vacations in Hawaii in January 2013 when he was 13 years old, we visited a place out in the ocean called Turtle Town, where a great many sea turtles lived. We were told, "Please don't swim to the turtles. Just be patient and wait, and they may come up to you. If they come up to you, please don't touch the turtles—just watch them." Of course, what does Johnny do? Swam toward the turtles AND touched them. I think he put patience because he WANTED to be more patient. He thought it was important and valued it. He said, "Patience is a very important virtue to practice, because if you expect immediate gratification from most things, often

you will leave disappointed." When he wanted something badly enough, he would wait for it until it happened, like the third time we tried to see Billy Joel and finally got to go.

3) Conviction — I was shocked in a pleasant way on this one because he used me as his example. I was so proud of him, and it turns out he was so proud of me. Johnny said, "I think conviction means showing confidence in what you believe in and know is the truth, and to stand by it. Though it may appear to be cliché and overdone, the biggest role model in my own life is my mother, Laura Stack. She is one of the most dedicated people I know to her profession, which is being an author and a speaker. She travels across the world, speaking about time productivity and using her books as references. She truly is the definition of a competent, assured professional, and she always believes in what she's doing. Her leadership skills that she's developed throughout her life have led her to where she is today and creating her own independently run business, The Productivity Pro, and being a symbol of conviction to me and many others." He never said this to me while he was alive. So, to all the parents out there, we never know the difference we are making in the lives of our children and the strong impact we can have on them.

4) Enthusiasm — Johnny had a huge enthusiasm for learning. He was scary smart and creative and curious and philosophical and loved to debate topics that were over my head. He always hated it when I bragged about him, but now he's gone, so I'm going to brag. He got a perfect SAT score in the math section, and a 34 on the ACT, to which he complained about the poor wording on some of the answers in the English section. He tutored our neighbor's daughter in math over one summer, and she was able to

test out of an entire year of math. He went to a camp at Stanford for a week to learn game design. He went to chess camps, robotics camps, and IDTech camps to learn various programming languages. He loved these experiences. He excelled in video games and was the highest rank in one of his favorites, CS:GO. In high school, his GPA was so high that after nearly failing the last semester of his senior year with four Ds when he was caught in the grip of addiction, he still graduated wearing honor cords.

5) Gratitude — Johnny wrote, "Simply put, expressing gratitude is showing you're thankful for what you have, or a kind act." When several of his friends came to visit the house over the last few days, they expressed their love for Johnny and shared memories with us. They showed us such kindness by taking the time to come talk with us. We tried to express gratitude in return by letting them pick something that reminded them of Johnny: a sweatshirt he wore, a stuffed Ram that was on the dash of his car, his special gaming headset, or his longboard. Johnny was right. Giving to someone else makes you feel good.

We hope that you can see through Johnny's Five Values how much he loved people and wanted to make a difference in this world.

You have all been so very supportive during this terrible time. We are forever grateful for these acts of service, your time, the cards and Facebook posts, the expense you went to, and mostly your prayers. You will never know how much everything has meant to us as we grieve. We have felt so comforted and surrounded by love."

After I spoke, Pastor Mark Shupe gave an inspiring, encouraging, and comforting message. Evan Dalrymple, who was Johnny's favorite singer from Cherry Hills Community Church, sang and was accompanied by Lance Garrett on the piano.

Afterward, guests gathered for lunch and beverages in the reception hall. They patiently waited for over two hours to greet and hug us and share their condolences. All in all, it was a wonderful, albeit exhausting, day that was also very healing. It provided our family and attendees with much-needed closure.

December 12, 2019 — Notes and Visits

Over the next few weeks, several of Johnny's friends visited and wrote. One came over to apologize for being the ringleader who got Johnny involved with marijuana in the first place. Another friend had taught him to longboard on the top deck of that garage and just needed to talk. The young woman Johnny got the curfew violation with came, as did the young man who used to be his best friend in youth group. I didn't know all of his friends who came over. All of them were grappling with the mystery of death and struggling with what went wrong. We loved on all of them, thanked them for being such an important part of Johnny's life, and reassured them they were not to blame.

I went through Johnny's texts and texted his friends from my phone (so as not to startle them) with the news. I didn't know most of them but thought they would want to know. I received this message back from a young lady who was in the second mental hospital with him:

I wanted to leave a note letting you know no matter what, Johnny LOVED all of you. As our friendship was formed in the hospital, Johnny ALWAYS talked about his family with sincere compassion. He said, "I made some poor choices." I told him to stay strong, that if he stayed on his meds regularly, he would see the benefit of them. (I am Bi-Polar with manic depression and personality disorder.) Johnny and I became fast friends. He always asked, "How do you smile when you're so sad?" My answer was a simple one. However, for Johnny, this was just starting. I tried to be supportive as a friend. After we were out and home, I called him a few times. At first, he was responsive and always ended with "We got this right?" and I said, "WE DO!!" I thought he was doing better. Then, I reached out to him and didn't hear anything. So, thank you for taking the time to let me know of Johnny's passing. I was broken for over a month. "I wish I would have" and "I should have" all ran through my mind. I am SO SORRY he chose this path. As a suicide survivor, I can tell you, he NEVER wanted to hurt you. We see it as stopping the pain. We don't see it as it is and what it does to the rest of the family. If I can offer anything to you, it would be that Johnny was a beautiful young man, just terribly lost. But he did love you very much.

Then we received a wonderful handwritten letter from a young woman who worked with Johnny. Here's an excerpt:

> I met Johnny on his first shift here at PetSmart. I work at the Banfield Pet Hospital, right next to the Pets Hotel. The first time I saw Johnny, he had the biggest smile on his face. I asked if he just got hired, and he said, 'Yeah, I'm so excited!' Even though I didn't work with him directly, I knew from that moment that he was going to be a wonderful coworker.

Every day, he would walk into work smiling. I honestly don't think I ever saw him without a smile on his face. That smile of his was so contagious, that if I close my eyes, I can picture it perfectly. He never walked by without stopping at my counter to say hi and ask how my day was going so far or how my weekend was. There was never a day he didn't smile, and there was never a day where he didn't say he was doing great. My heart hurts knowing that may not have been the truth. I only knew Johnny for a couple of months, but he made every day of them worth coming to work. He lifted everyone up with his high spirit and amazing energy. He'll forever be loved and missed, and his smile will never be forgotten.

The Psychiatric PA sent me a nice email. I was lamenting and asking her questions, and she responded:

Hi Laura, I read the journal entries, and it is apparent he was having paranoid delusions from the comments about UNC being a military base and the things about the mob and the whole world knowing about him. I genuinely believe that you did everything you could to help Johnny. It was obvious to me from the start that you were doing everything in your power to help. As I said before, taking Vraylar for one day would not have done much of anything. I am not sure why he decided to take the Vraylar that day since he refused for so long before. He could have had a glimpse that the delusions were not real. It was not because he didn't have a loving, supportive family. He had a lot of people trying to help him, but it was too late by the time he decided to really ask for help. I'm so sorry Laura. I really hope that you will eventually realize that you did everything you could and to not feel guilty.

I also wrote to the coroner after receiving his death certificate with SUICIDE written as the manner of death. I know she had seen hundreds of suicides, so I sent her Johnny's journals and asked for her opinion. I explained I was seeking expert opinions from anyone who could tell me what he was thinking at the time of his death and why he ultimately did it.

I was so pleased to receive this caring response:

Dearest Laura,

If I were a betting person, I would say he died from a deep schizophrenic episode. Every detail matters; his thoughts matter. Yes, Johnny was clearly, on the night of his death, delusional. He did not understand what he was about to do, because he couldn't. He could not understand that someday, the mental illness might clear. Someday, he might not be so tortured with episodes of circular thinking. Someday his racing mind would again take him to a ledge, but he should not jump. Was he delusional? Yes. Was it because he thought someone was chasing him? Yes. Who was chasing him? He was chasing himself.

What is most important, is not what his final communication was about, but that he communicated that he was clearly mentally ill. I know, without a doubt, your son did not rationally decide to take his life. This is the most important detail I ask you to hold closest to your heart. His journals were clearly delusional. The action was his delusional thinking (his brain), the reaction was to destroy his body; thus, shutting down his brain.

The communication is far too complex for us to know for sure his exact thoughts, but if you stay outside of the box and bring it to practical terms, he was mad and exhausted by his taunting and delusional brain. It's the only way he knew to shut it down. Mental illness is truly exhausting. Whether the illness was due to schizophrenia, bipolar, depression, drugs, alcohol, anger issues or any other maladies; these poor people are in deep turmoil.

According to a few very important comments from suicide survivors, they made arrangements, thought long and hard about what they wanted (suicide), but did not actually know for sure they would do it until by quick action, they followed through with their thoughts.

Did he know days in advance? Yes. Did he know that he would actually act? No. Hundreds of people get to the point of loading the weapon, standing on a ladder with a rope around their neck, or standing on a six-story parking garage, and they don't act. This tells us, that even though they are at the brink, they are never sure.

So, could you have saved him if you knew he was at the brink? No. Why? Because he could not tell you what he was even unsure about. Would he have told you if you loved him enough or loved him more? No. These people have so much love and attention around them, but they are still mentally ill. Love does not cure mental illness. Attention does not cure mental illness. A family's hypervigilance does not cure mental illness. So far, I know of no absolute cure, but he did, and he jumped.

Jill

After hearing from the Psychiatric PA and the coroner, I was sure Johnny had known he was going to do it days in advance—from the time he told us he wanted to go to church. He left his apartment with the intention of doing it. But he didn't know he would act until he saw that odometer. There was nothing I could have done to stop him at that point. He didn't reach out to me, and I didn't know where he was. I am so grateful all of these experts provided such comfort and perspective to help heal my broken heart.

December 20, 2019 — Signs of Suicide

After putting everything together a month after Johnny died, I realized he showed many signs of suicidality we may have missed. He was reaching out to loved ones, like his brother and sister, grandmother, and friends. He was trying to draw closer to God, suddenly wanting to go to church. He was making amends by telling me and John we were right about the marijuana. He was seeking drastic changes, such as wanting to move to California. He was making final arrangements in asking us what would happen to his dog. He was foreshadowing when he told me he wasn't going to take medicine for the rest of his life and wanted my permission to do it his way. Substance abuse and a previous attempt added to the danger.

My grief therapist assures me these incidents sounded like normal situations and conversation that no one would have picked up on. In hindsight, of course, we would have made different decisions had we known he would *die*. But that's illogical when you look at making decisions based on the information you had at the time. I will never fully, 100% understand why Johnny killed himself because I will never know what he was thinking at the time. But I have learned that you can't rationalize the irrational.

Could his death have been prevented? Who knows? It's complicated.
I do believe he lived longer than he otherwise would have because
he knew how much we loved him and tried to help him. There
were many times over the years I believe Johnny chose *not* to die
because of what we did for him. Ultimately, you can love your
children, but you can't keep them from dying if that is what they
choose to do. If love could have saved him, he would still be here.
We shouldn't be telling parents whose children died that "suicide
is preventable" or "there are always noticeable signs," because
that's not always true. The signs aren't always clear, and quite
a few people die by suicide who gave no sign. If there were signs
and you missed them, that doesn't make you a bad person, and
you shouldn't be ashamed. We just need to be more aware when
marijuana is in the picture.

So, if your child has been using marijuana and seems to be
struggling, how would you know if he or she is suicidal? I would
say there are some indicators or warning signs to watch for. We
developed the Johnny's Ambassadors C-A-R-E™ Model to help
you monitor these four areas:

1) Circumstances (life situations)

   ◆ Divorce of parents

   ◆ Breakup of relationship or rejection from love interest

   ◆ Rejection from peers or thinking they are unliked

   ◆ Bullying

   ◆ Failed a class or did poorly on a test

   ◆ Got in trouble with the law, parents, or school

2) Actions (behaviors)

   ◆ Giving treasured items away

   ◆ Reaching out to loved ones to say goodbye

- Suddenly wanting to be closer to God
- Isolating themselves from others and staying alone
- Suddenly stopping activities that previously gave them joy
- Relapsing into drug and alcohol use or increasing use
- Obtaining a gun or pills or the means to kill oneself

3) Remarks (words)
- "People would be better off without me."
- "I'm not going to be around to see it."
- "I'm done. I just want out."
- "I'm going to end it all."
- "I've decided to kill myself."
- "I'm tired of life."
- "What's the point of going on?"
- "Will it be like this forever?"

4) Emotions (feelings or indicators)
- Extreme sadness or crying
- Anger
- Sense of desperation for change
- Not sleeping enough or sleeping too much
- Uncharacteristically irritable or agitated
- Sudden mood changes
- Feeling hopeless or helpless
- Suddenly happy after period of sadness

If you see several of these indicators or if your child threatens suicide, it's important to ask, "Are you thinking about killing yourself? Are you considering suicide?" If your child hems and haws, then ask, "How serious are you on a scale of 1 to 10?" And then, "Do you have a plan?" If your child says anything about suicidality, take it seriously.

December 25, 2019 — Advice for the Grieving

It was nearing Christmas, and we were struggling with our grief. Many kind people reached out to check on us. Almost everyone expressed they were worried about saying the wrong thing or didn't know what to say. "There are no words to express . . ." was the mantra, but then they *did* express precisely what we needed to hear. Just knowing that people cared was comforting. It's nice to say to a grieving person, "I'm thinking of you," "How are you doing today?" or "I love you." Just knowing that someone cared enough to reach out is comforting.

Before Johnny's death, Christmas was our favorite time of year. After his death, we received many cards and emails from people who were also struggling with sadness and grief. It was enlightening to discover how many people don't feel so jolly during the holidays. My awareness and sensitivity levels have increased dramatically with this realization.

If you're grieving as well, you might try these tactics that helped me:

1) Remember what else you have to be grateful for. I have two other amazing children and a devoted, wonderful husband. I have a huge amount of support and friends who love me.

I'm grateful for the 19 years I had to enjoy our son beyond his mental illness. We acknowledge his struggles, but they don't define his spirit. Think of things you are grateful for on purpose.

2) Focus on positive things you can control. So much in life is out of your control, no matter what you do or try. Should have/could have/would have thinking creates negative thinking and guilt, so choose to focus on positive memories and experiences. Ask yourself, "Is this activity helping or harming me?" I didn't read the police report because that would harm me. I'm choosing to spend two hours reading sympathy cards because that helps me. I'm going to stop watching old Johnny videos and go to bed because that's not helping me right now. I'm giving away anything that creates negative memories. What can you do that makes you happy?

3) Attempt "normal" things. It might sound counter-intuitive, but it sometimes helped me to focus on other things. The last thing I wanted to do was put up the stockings and Christmas ornaments, but my children wanted it, and it helped us create a new, shared experience. Work a bit, meet friends, or go to a holiday party or Christmas show. Give yourself permission to leave early if you need to. All of these activities lifted my spirits. What can you do to distract yourself in a positive way?

4) Allow yourself to grieve. When a sound, situation, or item triggers sadness, let the wave wash over you and feel it. There is no timeline for this process. It's never going to be okay, but I'm going to be fine. How can you acknowledge your emotions as valid?

If you lost someone special to you, too, I wish you love and peace. If you lost a child to marijuana-related causes, please anonymously share your story at *https://johnnysambassadors.org/share*.

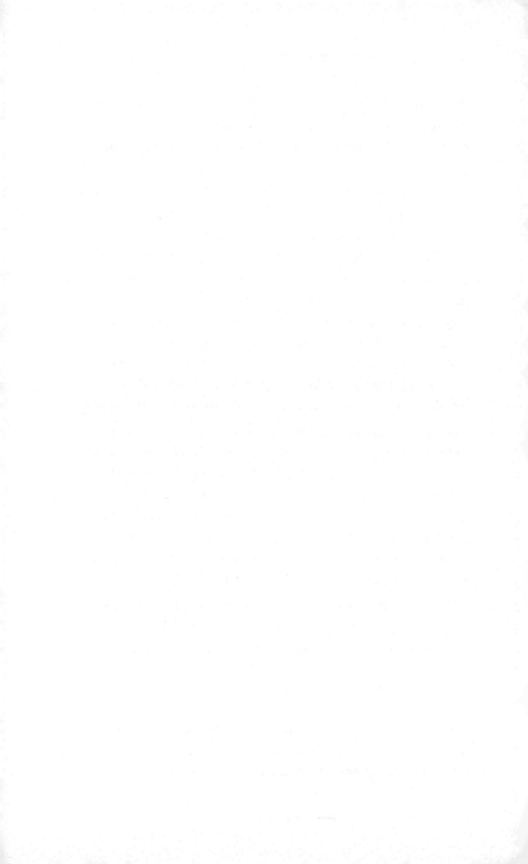

CHAPTER 9:

THE MISSION

January 1, 2020 — Lessons Learned

In the new year, I wrote several resolutions (more like reminders) for myself.

First, there's nothing I can do to change what happened. After the questions, guilt, whys, obsessive reading of Johnny's devices and journals, and what-should-I-have-done agonizing, Johnny is still gone. We actively worked on our grieving process. We attended a Parents of Children of Suicide group that we found extremely helpful. We participated in a program called GriefShare at a local church, first in person and then virtually when COVID hit. We found grief counselors to help us individually and as a couple. We attended a Survivors of Suicide (SOS) program at our local hospital. Caring friends sent me stacks of books to read. I wrote a lot and posted on Facebook, which was healing for me. I researched all I could about marijuana-induced psychosis. My lesson — *change what I CAN change.*

Second, I believe God knew this was going to happen, but He didn't cause it or allow it. It just happened. Johnny's death is no one's fault or responsibility. He was tormented by his mental demons, and in the end, he was exhausted by the struggle. It must have been awful, and I have a great sense of compassion for him. But no one forced Johnny to use marijuana, or withheld needed medications, or caused his death. Someday, I will understand God's plan for the good that will come from his death. My lesson — *I must let go of my anger at my inability to control what happened.*

Third, it's my responsibility to help others understand how Johnny died. I am determined to prevent any other parent from going through this agony. Insofar as I have the power to increase awareness, I can try to keep this from happening to someone else's child, if only they will listen with an open mind. No parent should ever feel this way. If a single precious life can be saved, that will be a potentially positive outcome to this horrible event. More important, helping someone else was Johnny's gift to the world, as he always sought to practice altruism. My new mantra is, "Forge ahead despite your pain and give meaning to your loss." My lesson — *helping others in someone else's name based on what he or she stood for gives you peace.*

Fourth, I must forgive, or it will eat me alive. When someone close to you has taken his or her life, a natural tendency is to seek understanding for the reasons it happened and then place blame. I did a lot of this at first. I blamed myself. I blamed the medical community. I blamed the insurance. I blamed Johnny's friends. I blamed Johnny. I blamed the marijuana. I blamed the marijuana profiteers. Then I realized that blaming was only making me bitter. My bitterness could not change what happened. It didn't resolve any issues; it blocked my healing.

Yes, I could blame all of these things, but I think the greater challenge to me was to forgive. I forgave myself and John for what I'm sure were things we did wrong or should have done differently. We did the best we could at the time with what we knew. We never gave up on him, and we never stopped trying to help him. That's the best we could have done. Of course, anyone would do things differently, looking back and knowing someone was going to die. But that's irrational thinking in the moment because people don't live their lives at every decision point wondering if someone will die if you do this. I forgave others who influenced his choices. I forgave Johnny for doing this to me. I forgave him for his poor choices. I forgave him for not listening to me. I forgave him for not taking his medicine. I forgave him for not letting us help him. He wasn't in his right mind. We recognize he was under the control of the THC, and it was no longer his fault. We forgave the insurance company, all of his doctors, ourselves, Johnny, and anyone else accountable *except* the marijuana industry. I DO blame this industry for creating the ridiculously high THC products that have no medical benefit to anyone. They only serve to make our children mentally ill. I blame the investors, the owners, the manufacturers, the legislators, and anyone else who contributed to making this poison available and thus taking my son away. That I can't forgive, and I will work to educate our legislators until potency caps and guardrails are in place to protect our young people. My lesson — *forgive those involved and do what I can to prevent others from making the same mistakes.*

Fifth, no one is immune from this happening—not even you reading this. Really crappy things happen to good people all the time. People look at my life and think it's perfect. *How could this happen to Laura?* Well, why *not* me? I'm not exempt from tragedy, and neither are you. Do you have any young adults in your life under 25 years old whose brains are still developing? It could happen to your children, your grandchildren, your nieces and nephews, or your loved ones. My lesson — *err on the side of being an annoying adult by warning the young people in my life. Keep talking about it and never stop.*

January 20, 2020 — Gifts and Regrets

On the two-month anniversary of Johnny's death, John and I attended a grief group for suicide survivors at our local hospital. The facilitator wanted to end "on a positive note" and asked us what gifts we've received or what good has come from our loved one's death. I thought that was a pretty daring, odd, and difficult question. Everyone looked at her blankly.

When it was my turn, I mumbled something generic like I was grateful for the people in this group who are willing to share their pain with strangers. But the question stuck with me, and I thought about it a *lot*. I was able to identify many gifts I've received as a result of Johnny's death.

If you're struggling with grief or loss, perhaps these will help you:

1) I've drawn closer to the Lord and have deeply experienced Psalm 34:18 which we printed on the wristbands we gave out at Johnny's memorial service, "The LORD is close to the brokenhearted and saves those who are crushed in spirit." I know Jesus has my son in his arms, and we will be together in the end with Johnny and Jesus in heaven. All is forgiven, and Johnny is healed. There's no greater comfort.

2) My family has drawn even closer in our grief. My husband John is my rock, and our two living children are my heart. Johnny will always be part of our family of five. We celebrated what would have been his 21st birthday with a party and cupcakes. He was an honorary groomsman in Meagan and Andrew's wedding.

3) We've experienced the extreme love and comfort of an incredible community of family, friends, clients, and colleagues, who have shown up for us in a big way and lifted our spirits with prayers, meals, gifts, donations, time, and cards.

4) An incredible army of friends, old and new, are helping us educate parents and teens about the dangers of today's high-THC marijuana on adolescent brain development, mental illness, and suicide. We are forming grassroots #StopDabbing teams at *stopdabbingwalk.com.*

5) Lives are being saved as we encourage parents and trusted adults to talk to their children about the harms of marijuana. We've developed a new online teen marijuana curriculum to share Johnny's story and educate them as a primary prevention strategy at *johnnysambassadors.org/curriculum.*

6) We've met incredible people in our new mission whom we otherwise wouldn't have met. We are blessed to make these connections and look forward to seeing what plans the Lord has in store. How will He make good come from Johnny's death?

While I have received many gifts from my son's death, I also have many regrets. I wish I would have been more educated about marijuana and taken more control when he was younger. I wish I could re-do the last three days of his life. Instead of begging him to take his medications on his last day, I wish I would have just held him and listened.

I always thought I knew what Johnny was doing, where he was, and who he was with, but looking back, I just didn't. I wanted to give him more freedom as he got older, but I should have been more in his business once I started seeing changes in his behavior.

He was always a fan of video games, but after the marijuana, there was a shift in how much time he spent alone that I didn't notice. Technology allows your children to hide things through features such as Snapchat's "My Eyes Only." When your child hits 16, you may be tired of parenting, but you have to keep at it. After working all day, you may not feel like you have the energy to deal with your teenager. I promise, if you were in my shoes right now, you *would* find the energy. Look at the time you have with your children. If you're not spending time with them as older teens, it may be time to get family counseling. When your children are talking to you, be laser focused on what they're saying. I wasn't a perfect parent, but I was a pretty good one. Johnny and I had a relationship that eroded over time, and I wish I would have made more purposeful attempts to regain it.

I regret my mindset. I thought it was all going to be better in the end. I thought, "He's a straight-A student, we're a Christian family, and he's just going through normal teen stuff, etc." I hoped he would get through this rough patch, and then everything would be okay.

I regret I didn't have more knowledge about dabs and today's high-potency marijuana. I only had the perspective of my own experiences in high school which were woefully out-of-date. Back then, it was basically Easter grass. I just didn't know. It wasn't until John and I went to CSU to clean out Johnny's dorm room that we found his nectar kit and said, "What the heck is this stuff?" We didn't even know those products existed. Your child will be offered marijuana at every high school and college party, so talk about it a lot. Today's marijuana isn't remotely the same as what we used to use.

I wish to God we would have known about home drug testing. I would have started early and made clean drug tests provisional for rewards and behavioral contracts. Drug testing would have given him the ability to tell his friends, "Sorry, I can't do that. My mom drug tests me."

I regret not sending him to a long-term, residential, dual-diagnosis rehab, recovery high school, or recovery community before he turned 18. One of the friends who got him involved with marijuana ended up going to rehab in Atlanta, and I remember Johnny talking about how messed up he was in the head. There was a very narrow window of time we could have done the same, and we missed it. When UNC wouldn't call the police or send him to a mental hospital, I regret not doing it myself. They moved him to a different dorm, and we didn't even know about it. I regret we didn't know about sober living housing. We would have tried something else versus a rental house after he turned 18.

(Note to parents: Make sure to get a medical or durable power of attorney and a HIPAA authorization for your children before they leave for college so you can help them in these instances. UNC wasn't prepared to handle cannabis-induced psychosis (CIP) and did the wrong things, the most egregious of which was not calling the police and/or having him admitted to a mental hospital.)

We had so many problems with insurance in Colorado. We had the one treatment center whose people wanted us to lie because Cigna, our insurance company, would not pay due to Johnny being addicted to "just marijuana." They told Johnny to lie and say he was also addicted to LSD, and he refused. At that point, I would have sent him out of state. We would have mortgaged our house—anything we needed to do, obviously. We were ignorant about the options and what to do. Once he turned 18, we lost all control. He withdrew consents with his doctor and psychiatrist, so I was in the dark. When he did get into a program, he checked himself out. When we did find a good program, he was actually shamed by the other participants for "just" being addicted to marijuana. They were cooler and tougher because they were addicted to crack and meth. Poor kid—he went to group and got teased for being weak-minded when he could have done circles around all of them intellectually. It shouldn't be so hard for a marijuana addict to get help.

I regret not asking him outright if he was suicidal. His first suicide attempt had been 14 months earlier, and maybe we let our guard down, thinking we were out of harm's way. Even his therapist, John Davis, said he didn't see any signs of suicide from Johnny and would have never suspected it. So, maybe we weren't as vigilant as we should have been. We just didn't know. I once told Johnny I was going to shackle myself to him 24/7 or duct tape him to the wall or chain him to his bed. Ultimately, you can't control others; they really have to want to get help. At that point, he refused the antipsychotics he needed, and he had a brain attack. It's no different than a heart attack. It's an illness.

Last, I regret I allowed our kids to taste alcohol at home before they turned 21. When I was growing up, we were allowed to have a small glass of wine with holiday dinners or join in the champagne toast for celebrations, so we did the same. If I had to do it over again, I would have insisted our kids not use any substances until 21, including nicotine and alcohol. They might have snuck it like many teens do, but at least I would have been providing a consistent message about avoiding any substance that affects the brain.

I wish I'd understood that any brief exposure to marijuana after sobriety causes relapse. I didn't recognize how hard Johnny was trying to be sober in the very end. He'd even given up nicotine and needed to put normal dopamine rewards back into his system. Not understanding the science, we didn't know how important getting him involved in jujitsu or another activity might have been to his recovery. He mentioned it one time in passing, but we didn't understand the importance of enrolling him.

Those are the things I regret. I just wish I would have loved him better somehow. Maybe any of the above would have changed the outcome, I don't know. I never will. But I hope Johnny's story changes the way you look at your children and your determination to connect with them. Johnny didn't feel like he could go on, and he chose not to have that conversation with me. We thought the suicidality had passed and got totally blindsided. When you're 19, you can't see that forever is forever, and you're not coming back like in CS:GO.

Remind your children that you love them, you are there for them, and you will be proud of them, even if they get a B.

February 7, 2020 — 20ᵗʰ Birthday in Maui

On what would have been Johnny's 20th birthday, we took our now-smaller family to Maui to scatter his ashes. We'd planned to take out an outrigger that morning, and our guides would have paddled us out into the ocean. Sadly, the winds were high that day, and we received a text message that our trip was canceled. We were so disappointed and spent much of the day wandering around, trying to figure out where to take his ashes.

Around 2:00 p.m., we thought we'd take a chance and walk over to the tour company office to see if the wind and waves had calmed down. I walked up to the operator, who was a full-blooded Hawaiian and had been doing outrigger tours all his life. His grandson now worked for his company. I was holding Johnny's ashes and told him about my son, that today was his birthday, and that we needed to find an alternative location. He looked at me, at the tube, out at the water, and then said, "Quick, let's go right now!"

We were thrilled! I sat in the back, and the operator's grandson sat behind me. John was in front of me and then James and Meagan. A second guide sat in the front. We went all the way out into the ocean. It was a bit choppy for my liking, but I was so happy to be out there. We each had flowers we'd purchased, and we dropped those into the water. I unscrewed the top of the tube and poured some ashes into the water. "Now you're back in your favorite place, my son," I said, crying. I handed the tube to John, and he poured out the rest. We all sat while the operator's grandson chanted and sang in Hawaiian as we watched the ashes travel down the waves with the flowers.

Just then, a humpback whale fully breached from the waves! And then another! I caught my breath and gasped. The grandson yelled and whooped and thanked the whales for welcoming Johnny. I grabbed my camera and caught the tail of one going into the water. They continued to jump and play around us for nearly five minutes afterward. It was so peaceful and healing.

When the whales moved on, we turned back to the shore (and gave a really nice tip to our guides).

Suddenly, it seemed that Johnny was everywhere. As we were leaving the beach, there was a hedge of Birds of Paradise growing right there—Johnny's favorite flower. Then, a stray black-and-white cat walked right in front of us and meowed. (Remember we always bought cat food for the strays and fed them.) We walked to get some ice cream and passed a clothes shop called—guess what—JOHNNY WAS. The window of the store had a Bird of Paradise with a hummingbird, our favorite. (I had a Hawaiian quilt commissioned after this incident with Birds of Paradise and hummingbirds.) Next, beautiful cloud formations formed in the shaped of an angel. You can see the photos on my Facebook page.[75]

I don't believe any of this was a coincidence—the whales, the flowers, the cat, the store, the clouds. All of it was from God to bring us comfort and clearly tell us Johnny was with Him.

February 20, 2020 — Godwinks

I've heard the Holy Spirit whisper to me on several occasions in my life, including when Johnny was born. I was told that Johnny would do something important in this world. Of course, I had no idea what it was, and I never heard anything else about it.

On Johnny's 5th birthday when I thought he was old enough to understand, I shared the "secret" with my young son. I told him, "God told me when you were born, you were going to do something really important in this world. We don't know what it is yet, but we are going to discover what it is together." Every time Johnny learned a new programming language, built a robot, or created the new operating system he called "Phoenix," he would ask me, "Do you think this is it, Mom?" We whispered about our "secret" repeatedly for many years so our other two children wouldn't know.

At the same time, I'd been speaking and writing for 30 years and was blessed with a fair level of influence with my platform, The Productivity Pro®.[76] I'd always prayed the Lord would show me how I could use my talents to advance the work of His Kingdom. I always thought it would be something related to women or mothers of preschoolers.

When Johnny died, I was confused because he had not done anything important in the world. I felt compelled to share what happened to him on Facebook so parents and teens would know about the dangers of high-THC pot. I wrote honestly in my posts about how the delusion and paranoia from the cannabis-induced psychosis had ultimately driven Johnny to kill himself. These posts were shared fairly well. I wondered if this was the important thing God had in mind for Johnny's life—teaching others about the harms of marijuana by sharing *his* story and *his* warning. I brushed it off, telling God this wasn't exactly what *I* had in mind, thank you very much. I said He would need to do something really, really obvious because I just didn't understand why Johnny had to be with Him.

The next day, I wrote a Facebook post[77] that asked people if they knew what "dabbing" was. *That post has been shared over 21,000 times.* I hadn't been able to reach that many people in all of my years in business with my own material. I'd never seen anything like that response!

God clearly told me, "Here is Johnny's very important mission in this world, and you are going to help him achieve what you talked about."

Well, I'm the stubborn type. This couldn't be it. How could Johnny have impact in this world when he isn't here? No, I don't want to. I'm too sad. I told Elizabeth Jeffries, my prayer warrior, what happened with the post going viral, and she told me to be obedient. So, I said, "Fine. I will go with the flow and do what He lays before me."

Well, that was all God needed. Never has anything been so easy. I visited my mentor, Dianna Booher, in Texas, and she told me about a nonprofit board she served on. She encouraged me to create the same kind of board with Johnny's Ambassadors. She and her husband Vernon were my first two board members, soon followed by Robin Thompson and Mellanie True Hills, both experts in the nonprofit space. I applied for our 501(c)3 status and received our acceptance letter within a month, which is a record for the IRS. A graphic designer, attorney, and accountant all agreed to help, pro bono, to get up and running.

I thought, "How in the world am I going to find time to start a nonprofit with two other businesses to run?" Then the COVID-19 pandemic happened, and all of my meetings and speaking business were canceled. So, with no work, I had a lot of time on my hands.

Dianna then introduced me to her book agent who connected me with Tom Freiling Publishing to publish Johnny's story because he believes the world needs to hear what happened. Next, 9News reached out and interviewed us, then ran a segment on teen suicide and marijuana (yes, it ran in Colorado twice now!). *The Epoch Times* published Johnny's story.[78] Parents shared stories on our website, saying, "Me, too!" I ran fundraisers, and the donations flowed in, allowing me to create an innovative online teen marijuana training and a weekly webinar series for parents. Robin Thompson told me these are all "Godwinks," and that nothing is a coincidence.

We started a Facebook group called Johnny's Ambassadors in ACTION which shares information about the harms of marijuana for youth. We also ask members to commit to demonstrating one of Johnny's five values in the community, workplace, or family. We started with 50 people, and we've now grown to over 1,200. Will you help me keep Johnny's spirit alive and be one of Johnny's Ambassadors? Please join our movement at *facebook.com/groups/ JohnnysAmbassadors*. Also register for our weekly newsletter at *johnnysambassadors.org/blog*. As I write this, we have over 2,000 ambassadors receiving our weekly newsletter which includes an educational article, the next webinar, and other announcements. We will soon be forming grassroots teams in cities around the world, so please keep in touch.

I have finally accepted the path God laid before me. Educating parents and teens about the dangers of today's high-THC marijuana on adolescent brain development, mental illness, and suicide is my God-ordained mission. Through Johnny's life and his warning, I pray many other youths will be saved from the harms of marijuana. I believe Johnny is doing something really important in this world after all.

February 21, 2020 — Eye Donor

After his death, Johnny created a living legacy of generosity with his ultimate gift of love–himself. His gifts included skin grafts, tendons and ligaments, corneas, and bones. There were several recipients of his soft tissue grafts around the U.S. Soft tissue grafts (ligaments and tendons) are transplanted to repair or replace damaged tissue or joints to help patients lead more active lives.

The Rocky Mountain Lions Eye Bank communicated with me when his healthy 19-year-old corneas were given, and I was able to write a letter to the donor recipient. I told her about the places Johnny's beautiful blue eyes had seen during his life and wished her a lifetime of seeing beautiful things through his corneas. They passed my note to her, and she wrote me back:

> Dear Laura, my name is Stella, I'm the married mother of 2 Adult Children, but also raised numerous Nieces & Nephews as my very own as well and the Grandmother (Unci) to many. I work as a Lakota Language Teacher and have been here for 28 yrs, and love my job especially all the children. I love spending time with Family & Friends, enjoy watching my family play darts, and watching Gossip Girl on Netflix. I too have similar traits and love selflessly, always giving to or helping others from my heart. I have always believed that one good thing, leads to many with kindness, respect, love & generosity. I will be forever grateful & appreciative for the gift of sight from your son. And I too have experienced the loss of my daughter, and I'm willing to help you in any way possible to lessen your grief. My continued prayers of Comfort & Strength will be with your Family & You always.

This letter is one of the most treasured blessings I've received from Johnny's death. In keeping Johnny's giving spirit of altruism alive, I encourage you to discuss organ, eye, and tissue donation today with those closest to you.

April 20, 2020 — 420 and 710 Days

Coincidentally, Johnny's five-month death anniversary was 420 Day. What? You don't know what 420 Day is? April 20, or 4/20, is International Weed Day, the day people around the world celebrate a drug that remains illegal in the U.S. 420 Day started in 1971 when a group of five teenagers would smoke weed every day at 4:20 p.m. after school before their parents got home. (You can read about the origins of 420 day here.[79])

Unbelievably, there are websites dedicated to helping people find all of the 420 events around the U.S. Denver Civic Center Park hosts the Mile High 420 Festival, an annual event run by the marijuana industry. They say the *"recommended" age is 18*, even though recreational marijuana is illegal for anyone under 21 in Colorado. So, many teens attended this event without their parents' knowledge, and your teens are happy that *you* don't know about it. While we're on the subject, do you know what 710 Day is? That's July 10, or 7/10, and is better known as Dab Day, which is OIL spelled upside down when you're high. The publication date of this book, July 10, 2021, is a symbolic anti-marijuana act.

If you're reading this, wrinkling your brow in confusion, and thinking, "What? I've never heard of 420 Day or 710 Day, and why does that matter to me? I'm 40 (50, 60, 70) years old and don't smoke marijuana." The point is that everyone under the age of 25 knows what 420 Day and 710 Day are. If you're a parent or grandparent or aunt or uncle with teens in your life, you must understand what this holiday is so you can discuss it with them intelligently when you hear the term. This isn't a "drug culture thing" or a "pro-pot" industry term. Most parents are in the dark. I was in the dark. I wish someone would have told me what 420 and 710 Days were. Moving forward, make sure you know where your teen is at 4:20 p.m. on April 20 and 7:10 p.m. on July 10.

CHAPTER 10:

THE RESEARCH

Let's Review —
How Can Marijuana Harm Your Child?

Here is a list of *some* of the things–all backed by scientific evidence–that could happen to your children if they use marijuana:

Chronic bronchitis symptoms[80]

Cannabinoid hyperemesis syndrome (CHS)[81]

Lung damage[82]

Heart disease[83]

Cancer[84]

Pregnancy complications[85]

EVALI[86]

Marijuana toxicity[87]

Brain damage[88]

Bipolar disorder[89]

Permanent loss of 6-8 IQ points[90]
Anxiety[91]
Panic attacks[92]
Depression[93]
Paranoia[94]
Psychosis[95]
Increased risk of schizophrenia[96]
Suicidal thought and behavior[97]

I highly recommend you read "The Effects of Cannabis Use on the Development of Adolescents and Young Adults"[98] from *The Annual Review of Developmental Psychology* (Hall et al. 2020). It is an overall review of all of the scientific effects of marijuana on youth, including dependence, brain function, other illicit drug use, psychosis, depression, anxiety, bipolar, suicidality, antisocial behavior, and the effects of legalization so far. Johnny's Ambassadors has also listed hundreds of scientific research studies at *johnnysambassadors.org/research*.

What's fascinating is these observations aren't new. In an article[99] published in the *New York Times* in 1971, doctors describe the harms to some of their young patients. These facts have been drowned out by legalization campaigns, trying to convince people that marijuana is "harmless." According to the National Center on Addiction and Substance Abuse (CASA) at Columbia University, 90% of Americans who meet the medical criteria for addiction started smoking, drinking, or using other drugs before the age of 18. Many kids will not use marijuana if they understand their parents oppose it. If you support marijuana use or are unclear about your stance, they will be more likely to use it. That means be extremely clear to communicate that you are against it.

What Are Cannabinoids, Exactly?

Cannabinoids are chemicals made by the cannabis plant. More than 80 cannabinoids have been identified, and they can affect how your brain and body function. The two most important cannabinoids are called tetrahydrocannabinol (THC), which is the most common, psychoactive cannabinoid in marijuana that makes users feel "high," and cannabidiol (CBD), which is the second-most common, non-intoxicating cannabinoid found in both marijuana and hemp plants. CBD doesn't make people feel high and is possibly helpful for controlling seizures and reducing inflammation.

Endocannabinoids are made by your body. They're made endogenously, or within the body, and some of them *act like* the cannabinoids from the cannabis plant. The two most important endocannabinoids are called anandamide and 2-AG, which stands for 2-acylglycerol.

Whether they come from plants or they're naturally made within your body, cannabinoid chemicals are like radio waves. They carry information like a messenger but need to land on an antenna for the message to be received. Receptors are like the body's antennas. Receptors are proteins that our cells make to detect the presence of these messenger molecules floating through the bloodstream or in the fluids that surround each cell. These endocannabinoid receptors are specifically tuned to pick up the signal from cannabinoid molecules and turn on. They are found throughout the brain and body, even in your digestive and reproductive systems.

How does THC work? It activates your endocannabinoid receptors throughout the body and brain and causes a high feeling. It's also responsible for the unpleasant feelings (like anxiety or paranoia) that some people report when they use marijuana. Because of human diversity, it affects different people in different ways. The body's endocannabinoid receptors can't tell the difference between fake and real cannabinoids, so that's why marijuana can affect how the body works. THC turns on the receptors designed to respond to your natural chemicals and blocks them. As a result, your body stops producing enough real chemicals.

Adolescent Brain Development

Adolescence is a time that combines a characteristic lack of judgment with a yet-undeveloped adolescent prefrontal cortex. This is a dangerous combination, considering marijuana is America's #1 most-used illicit drug and #2 most-popular substance after alcohol.

Marijuana severely affects adolescent health[100] during this critical time in these ways:

+ Problematic cannabis use typically peaks in adolescents, an age group that may be particularly vulnerable to its harmful effects.

+ Cannabis markets are dominated by high-potency cannabis (high THC, low CBD) with THC content steadily increasing worldwide.

+ Compared to low-potency cannabis, high-potency cannabis appears to be associated with a greater risk of psychotic symptoms, depression, anxiety, and cannabis dependence.

Mental Development in Adolescents

One of the tradeoffs of having big brains is that we humans
are born earlier than is optimal, leading to continued brain
development outside the womb. Brain development continues until
our mid- to late-20s. Like everything else, it kicks into high gear
during puberty, so kids ages 12 to 18 are at especially high risk for
anything that affects their physical and mental development. And
there's no doubt marijuana impacts mental development in young
people, which is also why it's illegal for recreational use until the
age of 21. The brain impact is even worse for 18-year-olds who get
"medical" cards (at least proponents acknowledge this science).

One study[101] of 45,000 Swedish military conscripts showed that
those who used marijuana more than 50 times before age 19
proved six times more likely to develop schizophrenia by age 34.

The mechanism causing these effects isn't entirely understood, but
repeated cannabis use in teens interferes with the development
of the prefrontal cortex,[102] the part of the brain directly behind
the forehead. This area of the brain, the last to develop, is
particularly active in adolescence because the brain prunes some
synaptic connections and firms up those most useful to survival.
Meanwhile, it refines its use of brain chemicals in preparation for
the transition to adulthood.[103]

Thus, the human brain goes through two major developmental
periods — one as a baby and one as an adolescent.

Picture your brain as a jungle. When you were born, your brain
was a tangled mess of vines consisting of about 100 billion
neurons. Your brain's first job is to grow and create *pathways*
through the jungle called neural circuits so you can find your way.

Next, your brain begins to close off pathways in the jungle you
rarely take in a process called *pruning*. Pruning helps our brains

learn and become more efficient. In other words, if you don't use those pathways, you lose them. Pruning basically keeps us from getting lost in the jungle, so it's a good thing. Heavy periods of pruning occur in your first two years of life and then again into your teenage years. It continues into your mid-to-late 20s.

Pruning happens through neurochemicals. As noted, one chemical in marijuana, THC, is called a cannabinoid. Our bodies also produce natural cannabinoids called *endo*cannabinoids, meaning internal. Anandamide is an example of an endocannabinoid. Our natural endocannabinoids have a similar molecular structure to marijuana cannabinoids—so similar that the brain has a hard time telling them apart.

One recent study from the University of Vermont[104] shows teen brain volume changes with even a small amount of cannabis use. The study published in *The Journal of Neuroscience* says gray matter volume *increases* when it's supposed to *decrease* during this time of pruning. "One possibility is they've actually disrupted that pruning process," senior author and University of Vermont (UVM) Professor of Psychiatry Hugh Garavan, Ph.D., said of the kids using marijuana. The study shows that even a small amount of cannabis use by teenagers is linked to differences in their brains. This research is the first to find evidence that an increase in gray matter volume[105] in certain parts of the adolescent brain[106] is a likely consequence of low-level marijuana use. "Consuming just one or two joints seems to change gray matter volumes in these young adolescents," Garavan said.

When you use marijuana, THC enters your brain and looks so similar to your body's own natural endocannabinoids that it fits right into your endocannabinoid receptors. Marijuana can disrupt the pruning process and accidentally change the way your brain develops in the future. It's like cutting your hair with your eyes closed—you might not get the results you expect. As a result, your brain may be less helpful to you when you're older. The UVM study looked at 46 kids who used cannabis only once or twice by the age of 14. Their brains showed more gray matter volume versus kids who didn't use marijuana which suggests the pruning process was disrupted. Key areas affected were the amygdala, which regulates emotion, and the hippocampus, which is involved in memory.

When you hit adolescence around ages 10 to 13, your brain takes the pathways that are left and makes them stronger in a process called *myelination*. Think of myelin as a thick cover around your nerve cells, like the insulation on an electrical wire. So, the activities you focus on regularly become permanent "superhighways" in the jungle. Myelin enables nerve cells to transmit information faster and allows for more complex brain processes. That means if you practice the piano frequently, learn a language, or throw a baseball repeatedly, your brain will "hard wire" that connection to make it easier for you to get better and repeat it. Similarly, if you use marijuana repeatedly, your brain "hard wires" that experience as well.

You want your child's brain pathways between cells to be strong like a steel bridge, not like toothpicks, and without potholes. If not, when they get older and put more weight on that pathway, it can break. Using marijuana just one or two times can have an effect on the developing brain!

The Impact of Marijuana on Your Brain
Let me point out five primary ways your brain is affected by marijuana use.

1) The Reward Circuit, regulated by the nucleus accumbens (we'll call it NAS) — A healthy brain rewards healthy

behaviors like exercising, eating, or hobbies. It does this by switching on the reward circuit and making you feel wonderful which then motivates you to repeat those behaviors. This part of the brain develops in early adolescence.

2) Emotion Processing, regulated by the amygdala (we'll call it AMY) — It's the "scout," always scanning the environment for anything important that might be a threat to you. Your amygdala is the warning system in your brain. It can make you feel happy or anxious.

3) Memory and Learning, regulated by the hippocampus (we'll call it HIPPO) — Your hippocampus is where you put all of the new things you learn to do.

4) Motivation and Drive, regulated by the orbitofrontal cortex (we'll call it OFC) — The OFC makes you want to get out of bed and do things.

5) Impulse Control and Decision Making, regulated by the prefrontal cortex (we'll call it PFC) — Your PFC allows you to say no to risky behaviors. The PFC is the last part of your brain to develop, so as a teen, you may act without thinking about the outcome. If you use marijuana regularly, the PFC doesn't develop further, making it difficult to control your impulses. It can be difficult to say no when your friends try to get you to use marijuana.

These five areas of your brain communicate using a neurotransmitter called glutamate. Here's how it works. When you use marijuana, THC enters your brain and clicks into your cannabinoid receptors located all over your brain. An abnormally high amount of the neurotransmitter dopamine is released to NAS, and it makes you feel good. NAS sends messages to the others via glutamate in these ways:

NAS says to AMY, "Hey, the next time you see that guy who gave us that marijuana, let me know."
NAS says to HIPPO, "Hey, the next time AMY sees that guy, remember what he is good for."
NAS says to OFC, "Hey, the next time AMY sees that guy, go get him because he has some good stuff."
NAS says to PFC, "Hey, don't worry about it—no one will catch us."

If you repeat this process a few times, it becomes hard-wired into your brain, and you never forget. Marijuana essentially hijacks the reward circuit in your brain. The THC molecules block your receptors, and your brain reduces the production of your own natural endocannabinoids. Your brain can no longer do its job correctly. It learns to crave more and more marijuana all the time to get those good feelings. Then you start needing more to keep from feeling bad, rather than because it feels good. When people can't stop using marijuana even when they want to, it is called addiction.

Teens who start using marijuana before their brains are fully developed will have permanent changes in their brain's structure and functioning. Working memory will be impaired, and they will be more impulsive, less attentive, less motivated, and slower to make decisions.

The Final Negative Influence
The problem here is getting young people to understand and actually worry about what might happen to them if they use marijuana. This is one of THC's most underestimated effects on adolescent brain development. Because teens don't understand how THC talks their bodies into betraying them, they don't see it as a major threat the way heroin or cocaine is. Worse, they use it because they consider it a low-risk gamble since "all of

my friends are using it." Most adults may think their kids don't understand the potential effects of early marijuana use, but in many cases, they do. They just aren't worried about anything happening to *them*. Teens feel invincible due to their PFC not being formed. They know that, unlike harder drugs, not everyone gets addicted to marijuana or has lingering effects. They also know it has a very low death toll.

One developmental neuroscientist Kuei Y. Tseng[107] often addresses young people about the negative effects of THC. He points out that all they *really* want to know is how much they can consume without harming their brains—something he can't quantify. Scientists have concluded there is no safe amount of marijuana during adolescent brain formation.

In an advisory released August 29, 2019, the U.S. Surgeon General went so far as to state, "until and unless more is known about the long-term impact, the safest choice for pregnant women and adolescents is not to use marijuana." Former U.S. Food and Drug Administration (FDA) commissioner Scott Gottlieb said he had significant concerns about the "great natural experiment we're conducting in this country by making THC widely available," citing his fears about "the impact that this has on developing brains."

Believe me, my son Johnny couldn't imagine it. He thought it would never happen to him. Those who have never experienced delusional thoughts that the mob is after you can't understand how awful it can be. Please don't risk finding out.

"Medical" Marijuana

Teens may have incorrectly heard that marijuana can help them get over negative things happening in their lives. Some people claim cannabis is a miracle drug with few negative effects; however, their claims are mostly wishful thinking and marketing tactics to get a new generation addicted to their products. It's important for you as a parent, grandparent, or loved one to understand the difference between short-term symptom relief and long-term problems caused by using marijuana. When you're educated, you can knowledgeably explain the dangers and get them proper medications, if needed, with a legitimate prescription.

Despite popular belief, it's rare for people to receive a real prescription for marijuana as medicine. If your teen were to receive an actual prescription, it would be in pill or liquid form, not weed you can smoke, dab, or eat.

Here are the cannabis-derived drugs[108] approved by the U.S. Food and Drug Administration (FDA):

* One cannabis-derived drug product called Epidiolex (cannabidiol) uses CBD only for two rare childhood seizure disorders.

* Three synthetic cannabis-related drug products include two dronabinol drugs (Marinol and Syndros) and nabilone (Cesamet) to treat nausea and vomiting caused by cancer treatments (chemotherapy). These use human-made THC, not plant-based THC.

These FDA-approved drugs are only available with a prescription from a licensed healthcare provider. The FDA has not approved any other cannabis, cannabis-derived, or cannabidiol (CBD) products currently available on the market as medicine. If my child had one of these disorders, I would be grateful this medicine could help them.

Dr. Ken Finn, a pain management specialist in Colorado Springs and one of Johnny's Ambassadors Scientific Advisory Board members, said, "The term 'medical' marijuana is a misnomer, because dispensary pot is not medicine; it's not 'prescribed'; it's 'recommended.' Any prescription for marijuana would be one of the FDA-approved medicines. Anything beyond those uses is considered 'off label.' Therefore, medical marijuana cards aren't prescriptions because they can't be filled at a pharmacy. Medications have to be purified and proven, and dispensary marijuana has failed the traditional definition of a 'medication.' If cannabis is to be considered 'medicine,' it should meet the rigors of scientific study. Unfortunately, 'medical' marijuana got a free pass at the expense of public health and safety. Products are frequently contaminated and poorly regulated. Additionally, Epidiolex, the only FDA-approved CBD, is not psychoactive, but it may cause liver damage, suicidal behavior and ideation, somnolence, and sedation." (Go to *epidiolex.com* and look under warnings and precautions.)

Additionally, numerous studies have concluded that smoking pot doesn't decrease pain[109] any better than taking a sugar pill. Others have shown that, at best, cannabis works about as well as codeine,[110] and some of the relief reported may result from the placebo effect.[111] On the other hand, cannabis use can increase pain sensitivity[112] for some kinds of traumatic pain when administered at high doses. As for glaucoma, the research shows cannabis decreases intraocular pressure in glaucoma patients,[113] but the effect lasts only three to four hours. The

American Academy of Ophthalmology disapproves of its use for glaucoma.[114] There are more effective treatments,[115] and you don't have to deal with drug crashes or addiction.

Even CBD lacks testing and regulation with many companies selling CBD products that contain very little CBD. Dr. Oz, heart surgeon, author, and host of The Dr. Oz Show, joined forces with Dr. Phil to investigate some companies fraudulently promoting CBD products using their names and images.[116] They asked Dr. Pedram Salimpour from a Los Angeles lab to test some of the samples, and they discovered one of the samples wasn't considered safe for human consumption due to elevated lead levels. It contained 15 times the safe level for lead. "Buying any of these products is like playing Russian Roulette," Dr. Phil said. For CBD products at this time, it's "buyer beware."

In time, researchers and pharmaceutical companies may approve new cannabis-related drugs for additional uses, but that time has not yet come. When it does, any new medicines will most likely be pills, liquids, or sprays, not recreational marijuana products such as dabs.

As of February 2021, the medication Sativex is undergoing FDA approval and has been available outside the U.S., including Canada and the UK. Sativex is a marijuana plant-derived drug with 2.7mg THC and 2.5mg CBD per dose. The National Academies of Sciences has used Sativex to support the use of cannabinoids for certain conditions such as pain and glaucoma. In this research, nothing above 10% THC in the plant has been studied, definitely not the 90%+ THC found in today's concentrates.

Medical marijuana dispensaries require a medical card for purchase of cannabis products in the 33 states (and District of

Columbia) where medical marijuana is legal. While it is illegal for teens to use marijuana recreationally until 21 years old, they try to get around it by getting a medical marijuana card at the age of 18. If they're over 18 and believe they need it for a self-diagnosed (or completely false, as in Johnny's case) "medical" purpose and a doctor agrees, they're in.

Teens can search online[117] for clinics near them that exist solely to provide users with medical marijuana cards. The marijuana exam fee costs $50 to $200 without insurance,[118] sometimes a bit more.[119] Once approved, the card is usually good for a year, although some states like Arizona have two-year cards.[120] A requirement to pay a fee to register a card varies by state.[121]

According to Colorado State Records of Medical Marijuana Cards as of November 2020, there are 131 med cards for children ages 0-10 years old, 140 med cards for teens ages 11-17 years old, and 3,900 med cards for young adults ages 18-20, which were given primarily for "severe pain." So, *on the one day* a teen turned from 17 to 18 years old, over 3,700 teens in Colorado developed a debilitating illness. This, of course, is ridiculous. Most teens like Johnny don't have any chronic conditions except wanting to get high. *Remember: No level of THC is safe for the developing brain.* Again, if you're the parent of a child with a rare seizure disorder who uses a legitimate prescription for a cannabis-derived product, this conversation doesn't apply to you, and I'm glad it's helping your child.

Sadly, medical marijuana cards are hardly the cure-all teens might think. They believe this "medicine" will treat their stress or anxiety. Yes, getting high may make them temporarily forget their problems and help them "chill out" in the short term. However, it doesn't fix their problems; it just means they don't care for a while. Marijuana isn't medicine—it's numbness. The issues remain when they come down off their highs. Teens may feel good when first trying it (if they don't experience psychosis), but those happy feelings are short-lived. In the long term, marijuana may create the very problems they are trying to avoid. And some young people will experience psychotic symptoms and suicidal ideation, just like Johnny did. We do not know which kids will be affected, so I believe it's just not worth the risk.

You may be thinking, "Wait, didn't our ancestors use marijuana for supposed medical reasons?" Yes, but just because some groups have reportedly used marijuana to treat pain and other maladies since ancient times, it doesn't mean we don't have more effective treatments now which don't carry the same risks of harm as marijuana does.

It Gets Worse

Teens may perceive marijuana may help them "chill out" if they are feeling anxious, but marijuana will cause them to feel MORE anxious in the long term.[122] In fact, marijuana use is quite dangerous for adolescent brain development and mental health. We know for certain that cannabis use can cause severe psychological and physical effects in both the short and long term. This is especially true for modern cannabis, which may contain up to 90-99% THC. Effects that don't typically lead to contacting your family physician for help start with compromised judgment,[123] permanently lowered IQ,[124] and loss of motivation[125] but can scale up to anxiety (including panic attacks between uses, often due to cannabis-induced anxiety disorder), depression, psychosis, paranoia, and a much greater risk for schizophrenia and suicidal thoughts and behavior in the long term. Too much marijuana is simply poisonous. Marijuana toxicity causes nausea, vomiting, panic, anxiety, high blood pressure, confusion, and most of the other symptoms some people seek to treat with medical marijuana.

Don't Fall for It

It might surprise you to learn that some teens don't use marijuana to get high. In a number of small studies,[126] teenage users have reported using marijuana primarily to cope with life issues. The symptoms they most often target include physical pain, anxiety, depression, ADHD, grief, and stress. Others reported using it to help them sleep or concentrate; the latter would dovetail with the ADHD and, potentially, depression and anxiety issues. Some use pot to help relieve more than one symptom.

Often, these teens know about *some* of the negative effects of pot, including loss of concentration and a decreased ability to learn. But they claim they don't use the drug in excess, and that, in fact, their usage is "normal."[127] Clearly, they feel its benefits outweigh its costs and deliberately limit their use to avoid addiction and mental illness. Unfortunately, these young users aren't sufficiently informed to properly regulate, or "titrate" in medical terms, their drug use. As a result, sometimes the self-medication results in addiction or a worsening of the very symptoms they're trying to alleviate.

Note that these are *not* teens who have been diagnosed with ailments like seizures, cancer, or glaucoma for which the medical use of marijuana[128] has been approved. They've made the decision to medicate themselves with the drug under recreational use—that is, they do not have med cards, and it has not been prescribed for them. This is made simpler by the fact that marijuana products are easy to acquire, even for underage buyers. (A 16-year-old Colorado teen I just talked with said any high schooler can get marijuana in five minutes.)

Many users claim marijuana helps them relax and temporarily forget their symptoms, but the scientific evidence for that is lacking. Much of the anecdotal evidence contradicts this idea as well. Marijuana use does not aid in concentration, and for many users, it stimulates them rather than makes them sleepy due to the high THC content of most modern marijuana products.

Especially with high THC potency, users can end up with worse effects than those they're trying to escape, including heightened anxiety (e.g., cannabis-induced anxiety disorder), psychotic breaks, paranoia, deep depression, and schizophrenia (up to five times the normal rate). It may also trigger suicidal tendencies and thoughts (up to seven times the normal rate[129]). In one study of twins, marijuana use was associated with twice the normal risk for depression.[130] The scientific evidence shows that in most cases, anxiety actually increases between uses[131] and may scale up to outright panic. Such attacks can occur even while using.[132]

Using marijuana for anxiety and depression is like walking a high wire over a pit of razor blades without a net. It's best to see a psychiatrist and get evaluated for an FDA-approved prescription to help manage anxiety and depression and not self-medicate with marijuana.

As far as I could find in my research, there have been no peer-reviewed scientific studies or trials that show any *positive* effects of marijuana use on adolescent or public health. For example, has there been:

- Decreased adolescent use and addiction?
- Decreased hospital utilization, particularly with youth?
- Decreased opioid and other drug-related overdose deaths?
- Decreased psychiatric episodes?

- Decreased suicidality?
- Decreased marijuana-related driving fatalities?
- Decreased marijuana DUIs?
- Decreased cancer?
- Decreased crime?
- Decreased drug cartel activity?
- Increased vocational wealth and graduation rates?
- Increased healthy baby births when used during pregnancy?
- Increased IQ with chronic use?

Can anyone in the marijuana industry provide any of these studies? No, because they don't exist. My search indicates there is *no* validated research on the high-potency THC products available in dispensaries today that indicates they are advantageous for anything medical or even safe for anyone. However, the opposite of all of these statements has been scientifically proven to be true. So, if there is no regulatory oversight for health, safety, or efficacy, how can these products be considered "medical"?

When you get right down to it, self-medicating with cannabis is dangerous, especially for adolescents, and it doesn't work all that well anyway. With rare exceptions, there's always a long-term, legal medication or therapy that works better for all of the symptoms discussed here. If you think otherwise, you're fooling yourself and flirting with dependence, addiction, and mental illness.

Teens may be able to find a doctor willing to give them med cards if they are over 18. A doctor may honestly believe cannabis with THC content has medicinal effects for anxiety or stress, for example, but such views aren't supported by significant scientific proof or FDA approval. If your teen's "medicine" contains THC, it isn't medicine. It arrests the development of the adolescent mind until it's fully formed in the mid-to-late 20s. You wouldn't go buy your child a bottle of vodka to help them with stress, would you? By now, I hope you realize the best way to help a child with psychological problems is to take him or her to a licensed psychiatrist for a federally approved medication or treatment, not to a medical marijuana doctor for marijuana.

Marijuana, Psychosis, and Schizophrenia

There are hundreds of peer-reviewed, scientific articles that show a correlation between marijuana use and psychotic outcomes such as schizophrenia (too numerous to list here). The question of whether marijuana is causal for psychosis has been answered in the affirmative by applying standard principles of causation used in pharmacological and epidemiological research.

There are identical twin studies, such as in the work, "A Polygenic Theory of Schizophrenia" by Irving I. Gottesman and James Shields in 1967, in which one twin gets schizophrenia and the other does not. That tells us it is not purely genetic because there are many environmental factors involved, including marijuana usage. Even if Johnny had been genetically predisposed, it's not a sure thing he would have gotten schizophrenia.

THC causes psychosis even in instances of NO mental illness. A study done in Great Britain[133] gave light users of marijuana with *no* family history of mental illness a moderate THC dose, and 40% of them exhibited psychotic symptoms.

Research comparing the mental health effects when low-potency cannabis was available versus when high-potency cannabis was available found a greater proportion of initial onset psychosis cases being attributed to cannabis use. In addition, a study published in the Lancet[134] compared 900 people from Europe and Brazil who had been treated for psychosis with 1,200 people who had not. Both groups were surveyed on a host of factors, including their use of marijuana and other drugs. The study's authors concluded that "people who smoked marijuana on a daily basis were three times more likely to be diagnosed with psychosis compared with people who never used the drug. For those who used high-potency marijuana daily, the risk jumped to nearly five times."

Dr. Erik Messamore, one of Johnny's Ambassadors Scientific Advisory Board members, wrote the following:[135]

Emerging scientific findings are more supportive of a causal relationship — that regular cannabis use actually drives the extra schizophrenia risk. The anandamide-depletion hypothesis can explain how regular cannabis makes schizophrenia more likely.

The hypothesis is based on findings that:

- Inflammation is a major contributor to psychosis.

- The brain's own cannabinoid substance, anandamide, rises during inflammation and is part of a natural anti-inflammatory response.

- Regular exposure to plant-derived cannabinoids reduces the brain's ability to produce its own cannabinoids.

This would make the frequent marijuana user more vulnerable to the effects of brain inflammation and thus more prone to develop a schizophrenia-like psychosis.

Marco Colizzi and Dr. Robin Murray stated in the *British Journal of Psychiatry*:[136]

> "It is now incontrovertible that heavy use of cannabis increases the risk of psychosis. There is a dose-response relationship, and high-potency preparations and synthetic cannabinoids carry the greatest risk." Colizzi wrote, "Patients do not start using cannabis to self-medicate their psychotic or prodromal symptoms or side-effects of drugs, but rather use it for the same reasons as the rest of the population, principally for its 'high.' The risk of psychosis remains after controlling for personality disorder and use of other psychotogenic drugs. Some overlap between genes carrying susceptibility to schizophrenia and to drug use has been reported but insufficient to explain more than a fraction of the relationship. Of course, the vast majority of people using cannabis do not develop a psychotic disorder. Not surprisingly, people with a paranoid or 'psychosis-prone' personality are especially vulnerable, alongside people with other risk factors for psychosis such as childhood trauma. Starting use in adolescence and having a family history of psychosis also carry more risk; some evidence points to variants of genes involved in the dopamine system conveying susceptibility."

Be aware these studies address risks that can be clearly seen only by looking at large numbers of people. That is, as a group, adolescents exposed to THC, particularly more potent THC, have a higher probability of developing schizophrenia. That doesn't mean every kid who uses marijuana will get schizophrenia. Yet, because you don't know in advance how your 14-year-old will respond (no one does), you are being a responsible parent by telling them, "Don't dab because you're more likely to get schizophrenia."

Johnny didn't have psychosis before using marijuana or with any other drug he tried. It was only after a lengthy period of high-frequency use of high-potency wax that he had mental breaks. A study by Grewal and George in the *Psychiatric Times*[137] showed eight distinguishing features between idiopathic (genetic) psychosis (e.g., schizophrenia) versus cannabis-induced psychosis (CIP).

The fact that Johnny experimented with LSD on occasion also doesn't indicate that's what gave him schizophrenia. Two large studies in Scandinavia have shown that LSD is less likely to lead to schizophrenia spectrum disorders over time than is marijuana (Niemi-Pynttari et al., 2013[138]; Starzer et al., 2017[139]). In addition, there are important ways in which the effects of LSD and marijuana differ that are relevant to what happens when someone has schizophrenia.

Dr. Christine Miller told me this via email:

> Marijuana usually does not cause classic visual hallucinations the way that LSD does, which can cause users to see objects in spaces that are actually empty (pink elephants flying around an empty room). Usually, the hallucinations with marijuana-induced psychosis are auditory, and when the visual system is perturbed, it may be a perturbation of the significance attached to what someone is seeing, i.e., a visual 'illusion' (King et al[140]). So, for example, someone with marijuana-induced psychosis may think they are seeing dead people passing by in cars, and there are really cars passing by, but the people inside them are not dead. Read the study to understand the difference between illusions and hallucinations.

> This difference between LSD and marijuana is important because it is also consistent with marijuana-induced psychosis being closer to schizophrenia than LSD-induced

psychosis. In classic schizophrenia, the hallucinations are predominantly auditory (only 27% are reported to experience visual hallucinations and in some of those studies, they may not have distinguished hallucinations from illusions). Unlike LSD, administration of marijuana to mentally healthy subjects in the clinic elicits visual illusions not hallucinations (Vadhan et al.[141]), and administration of marijuana to individuals with a psychotic disorder elicits predominantly auditory hallucinations (Henquet et al.[142]).

Marijuana Leads to Other Drug Use

Every other year since 1991, the Centers for Disease Control and Prevention (CDC) conducted a study of youth behavior[143] in six significant categories with the intention of monitoring and managing negative behavior. One of the categories they monitor is "Alcohol and Other Drug Use."

The Youth Risk Behavior Surveillance System (YRBSS)[144] last monitored these categories in 2019 with a series of "national, state, territorial, tribal government, and local school-based surveys of representative samples of 9th through 12th grade students"[145] in conjunction with a larger sample of middle school students[146] from a small number of interested localities. The adolescents involved were ages 13 to 17.

During each survey, students self-report their behavior on pencil-and-paper questionnaires completed during a single class period. About 4.9 million high school students have completed the questionnaire since 1991. The CDC has estimated the reliability of the questionnaire as good, though they note that students tend to under-report their weights and over-report their heights. In 2019, the YBRSS received 13,677 usable questionnaires from high school students from almost every community in the country and more than 83,000 from middle schoolers in selected cities, states, and territories.

Here are some data points from the high school group:

- 36.8% reported lifetime marijuana use.
- 21.7% reported current use (17.1% of ninth and tenth graders and 26.6% of eleventh and twelfth graders).
- There were no significant differences in use between boys and girls.
- Asian-Americans had the lowest rate of use at 14.7%; Native Americans topped the list with 48.3%.
- An average of 5.6% of students reported using marijuana before age 13.

While that data may be startling, the most troubling factor to rise out of it was the *association between teen marijuana use and prescription opioid misuse*: HAVING EVER USED marijuana was the *top* co-occurring substance use behavior for high school teens who have abused opioids in the past 30 days, even OVER ALCOHOL use in the past 30 days.

Let that sink in—*marijuana is now the biggest gateway drug.* Whether a high schooler has *ever* used marijuana in the past is the most common behavior of those who abused opioids in the most recent 30-day period.

Dr. Kevin Sabet, who wrote the foreword to this book, is president of Smart Approaches to Marijuana (SAM) and a former three-time White House drug policy advisor. He said, "This survey confirms a trend we have been noticing: every other drug among young people is going down with the exception of marijuana…we have to understand that drug use does not happen in a vacuum—co-use is a real phenomenon."

Two other scientific studies confirm this. In the first one, "Probability and Predictors of the Cannabis Gateway Effect: A National Study,"[147] 6,624 individuals were studied who started cannabis use before any other drug. The authors concluded, "Lifetime cumulative probability estimates indicated that 44.7% of individuals with lifetime cannabis use progressed to other illicit drug use at some time in their lives." The second study, "Patterns of Cannabis Use During Adolescence and Their Association with Harmful Substance Use Behaviour: Findings from a UK Birth Cohort,"[148] sought to assess cannabis use among 5,315 UK teenagers ages 13-18 years and its influence on problematic substance abuse at the age of 21. The authors noted, "Sex, mother's substance use, and child's tobacco use, alcohol consumption and conduct problems were strongly associated with cannabis use." The authors further concluded, "One-fifth of the adolescents in our sample followed a pattern of occasional or regular cannabis use, and these young people were more likely to progress to harmful substance use behaviours in early adulthood."

Discouraging marijuana use, then, should help discourage other drug behaviors. While this may seem obvious, a growing false assumption is that marijuana is not a dangerous drug for children because, hey, we did it when we were kids. Understand that today's marijuana is HIGHLY POTENT, and many marijuana products have the raw THC extracted into dabs, shatters, and waxes. Children and their developing young minds are highly vulnerable to marijuana use.

Just because marijuana grows out of the earth doesn't make it safe. Many other growing things are toxic, including deadly nightshade, oleander, and poison ivy. Some plants like poppies are made into drugs. Rattlesnakes and arsenic are natural, too.

The CDC report states, "Specifically, the high rates of co-occurring substance use, especially alcohol and marijuana use, among students currently misusing prescription opioids highlights the importance of prevention efforts that focus on general substance use risk and protective factors."

Clearly, it's time to step up our anti-marijuana programs and activities, starting at younger ages and striking hardest in minority communities.

Talking to Your Kids

As parents, you and your partner are your child's first and most important teachers. They pick up just about everything from you—from speech to basic habits to attitudes. No one will shape their young minds more. This gives you the opportunity to create a solid foundation for your child's mental health.

When you're there for your kids, they'll always look to you for advice and see you as a role model. The National Surveys on Drug Use and Health (NSDUH), which are conducted by the Substance Abuse and Mental Health Services Administration (SAMSHA), analyzed data from 2015 through 2018. The researchers focused on adolescents and young adults who had a parent born between 1955 and 1984. Parents also took part in the survey. Researchers found that kids with mothers who had used marijuana in the past but not for at least a year were 30% more likely to use marijuana compared to kids with mothers had who never used the drug. Compared with kids whose mothers never used marijuana, those whose mothers used the drug within the past year were 70% more likely to have started using cannabis. Similarly, kids with fathers who used marijuana within the past year were 80% more likely to use cannabis compared to kids whose parents never used the drug.

Normalizing marijuana through commercialization and legalization means, as a parent, there is no neutral response to marijuana anymore. A neutral or non-response is effectively *pro-pot*; only a clear rebuff or refute is *anti-pot*. So, take advantage of this and talk with them on the overall harm of marijuana on their mental health, especially today's more potent extract forms.

No matter how young or old your kids are, keep the following advice in mind when it comes to talking about substance abuse.

First, don't assume your kids already know the risks. They may not, especially when the media, friends, and movies try to make drug use look cool. They need to know why they should "just say no," or you're going to get pushback. So, educate yourself by reading the research compiled for you on our website at *johnnysambassadors.org/research*.

Second, quantity has a quality of its own. People talk about spending quality time with their kids, and that's important. But quantity time is just as important when it comes to building emotional ties, especially when you talk about your lives together. A Columbia University study[149] concluded that young people are less likely to drink or use drugs when they eat at least five meals a week with their families. Take advantage of times like this and car rides, vacations, and more to talk.

Third, when talking to your kids about drugs, broaden the subject as they become capable of understanding more. Include other types of substance abuse such as smoking, drinking, and hard drugs.

How to Begin

Begin talking with your kids about drugs when they are young[150] (some experts recommend as young as five years old or even younger) and repeat the conversations regularly. Make them two-way conversations, not one-sided lectures. Let your kids talk and ask questions. Let them know you're discussing this stuff because you love them and don't want them to get hurt.

If your kids feel like they can ask you questions about drugs and depend on you to give them straight answers without yelling or condemnation, they're more likely to come to you for advice when drug use raises its ugly head.

Like a Booster Shot!

Luckily, most kids don't do drugs. One reason is that most of the time, kids actually listen to their parents. So, talk to your kids about drugs! Think of it as another type of booster shot to fight off an especially nasty virus. This is one conversation to have repeatedly as your kids' lives (and the rest of the world) change. You want what you've said to stick and hope it will.

My father was a colonel in the U.S. Air Force, so I was familiar with the role of a drill sergeant teaching recruits something over and over until they do it automatically. Of course, you won't be harsh like a drill instructor, but when you repeat yourself, your kids will hopefully reject drugs automatically.

Young Children

Like so many important topics, it's hard to pinpoint the perfect time to have "The Drug Talk" with your kids. You don't need to worry about the tiny tots since they're rarely out of an adult's supervision. But many experts suggest you begin talking to your kids about drugs when they are fairly young. According to some, starting in preschool[151] isn't too soon.

Starting early is a great way to make openly discussing drugs and their damaging effects part of your kids' normal life experience. If you've talked to them about drugs for as long as they can remember, it won't seem odd when you bring up the topic again to warn them of a new threat or when you expand the discussion to include other forms of substance abuse.

Wait until your kids are old enough to understand the basics, but don't put off the first drug talk past age ten. That's when they're still young enough to trust you about everything and will listen. This changes soon enough, believe me!

Make your drug talks more than a series of stern warnings. The conversations should be informal, back-and-forth conversations. Tell your kids *why* drugs are bad for them, especially that it hurts their brains which are supposed to get smarter and smarter as they get older. Drugs keep their brains from getting smarter. Let them ask questions and ask a few yourself until you're sure they understand. You want to keep them safe, so let them feel that.

You could begin by talking about simpler drugs, such as over-the-counter and prescription drugs. Ask your kids what they know about medicine and how it's used. Explain that these drugs, while legal, are so strong that a doctor must decide whether someone needs them. Plus, there are limits on how much should be used, or they can make people feel bad.

Also point out that if they must take medicine because they are sick, they shouldn't let a friend use it. If friends are taking a certain medication, tell your child not to use theirs either. And they should NEVER use your prescriptions. Those are meant for grownups and might make them sick, both in the body and in the head.

This is also a good time to start discussing alcohol use and how beer, wine, liquor, etc., are meant only for grownups. As before, ask what they know about alcohol and check to see if they have any questions. Bring up alcohol poisoning and explain how it can hurt their bodies and brains. Talk about smoking being bad for your heart and lungs and marijuana being bad for your brain—and your life.

Obviously, be extremely careful if YOU are bringing legalized cannabis in various forms into your home, including edibles such as candy, snacks, and ice cream. I would encourage you to stop using marijuana yourself so you aren't setting the wrong example for them.

Tweens
Back when I was a kid, nobody had ever heard of the term "tween." Basically, you were a baby, a toddler, a preteen, or an adolescent. Oh, a few people had used similar terms as early as the 1920s, and Tolkien applied it to hobbits in 1954. But as it exists today, it's a marketing term that appeared in the late '80s and became popular in the '90s. It refers specifically to kids who are no longer children but not yet teenagers—that is, those from the ages of nine to twelve.

And boy, ever since it became a marketing category, everyone from fashion designers to drug dealers have heavily marketed to the tween demographic.

During their tweens, kids start to tune in to social differences and the culture around them. Not that little kids don't fall prey to such things; anyone who's had a kid see a toy on TV and exclaim, "I want one of those!" knows better. But puberty often starts in the tweens, bringing everything into sharper focus.

Your tween may not have gotten there yet, but plenty of other kids in their social circles have, and *their* behavior will inevitably affect your tween's behavior. It's kind of a ripple effect with stronger tweens representing the thrown stones that roil the surface of a still pond.

Even if their hormones haven't begun raging, your kids may experience teasing, bullying, isolation, cliquish behavior from others, and other blows to their self-esteem. Then there's the pressure to fit in as they learn about drugs, sex, and other influences from their peers. As a result, your tween may start looking away from you as life's guideposts and widen their circle of role models, some of whom may not be a positive influence.

Something I regret not doing better was monitoring who Johnny was hanging out with. These days, it's more important than ever to keep an eye on the crowd your tween children hang out with. Be especially alert to changes in their circle of friends. Allegiances will change; some friends may fade into the background while others become more prominent. Discuss these changes with them. Know where your kids are when they're not at home and know who they're with. In hindsight, I would have insisted on knowing friends' parents and their addresses. It's hard to admit these things now, but it's important to help others learn from my mistakes.

It's also time to set strict boundaries and expectations regarding their behavior, including anything drug or alcohol related. It turns out Johnny was leaving the house late at night, so I highly recommend installing a security system (like the one we now have) so you can tell if a door or garage was opened. If you've already been having these talks, your kids know what you expect of them in this regard. When they become teens, ensure there are *no surprises* about your expectations of behavior and *zero tolerance* for alcohol and drugs.

You may be wondering how often to have drug talks with your tweens. I recommend a discussion by the age of 10 for sure. It's easiest to do as you watch a television show where drugs are involved (especially one that normalizes marijuana or casually shows people smoking) or when you drive to an event or practice and see a sign. Just chat with your child often about your lives and expectations—not just when something bad happens. A good time to do this is at the dinner table. As mentioned, kids who eat with their families five or more times a week are less likely to abuse drugs or alcohol than those who don't.[152]

By this point, your kids probably understand how dangerous prescription drugs can be when used improperly but remind them occasionally anyway. Expand your discussions to include new threats as they appear. Even if cannabis is not legalized for recreational use in your state, discuss the dangers cannabis edibles and highly concentrated THC products like dabs or wax can have on their minds. Share the extensive research we've gathered on our website at *johnnysambassadors.org*.

In middle school, opportunities for drug and alcohol use may arise as your tweens test their boundaries and prepare for what they think adulthood will be, so make your drug conversations more serious. Discuss the challenges of peer pressure and how to fight it. Use examples of people they know, including friends, family members, or celebrities whose lives have been damaged by substance abuse. Give ideas for better coping mechanisms and help your child engage in healthy activities. Model appropriate stress relief that does *not* include alcohol and drugs. Don't use alcohol frequently whenever something good happens or you are stressed out. Identify and teach healthy coping strategies, including exercise, team sports, karate, horseback riding, taking a bath, getting a massage, walking your dog, or praying—to name a few.

If your kids ask if you've ever used drugs (and they probably will), answer honestly but do not expand on any of your exploits. Let them know how different today's marijuana is than when you smoked it and why it's important not to do it.[153] If you had a substance abuse problem, tell them how hard it was to escape it. Emphasize that you'll never let it happen again, and invite them to learn from your mistakes.

Heavily emphasize the fact that drugs damage their brains because they are still developing. Remind tweens their brains won't stop developing until their mid-to-late 20s. Until then, any drug use, even a little, can cripple their mental development and even cause mental illness.[154] High-dosage cannabis products could even make them psychotic or paranoid.[155]

Try approaching the subject from different angles so your child won't get bored with the repetition and tune you out. For example, in one talk, you might want to warn them about how drinking alcohol can severely damage brain cells, making it harder for them to transmit signals[156] (and therefore thoughts) in the brain. Excess consumption can even kill brain cells, permanently damaging memory and the body's ability to regulate its temperature and lower the heart rate. The amount of alcohol required to cause such damage is lower for them than for an adult. All it takes is half the average adult amount, which doesn't amount to much anyway.

Teens

If there is ever a time when parents struggle with their children, it's during their teenage years. Not all teens rebel, but many have their share of clashes. After all, they know just enough about life not to know what they don't know.

As Mark Twain once put it, "When I was a boy of 14, my father was so ignorant I could hardly stand to have the old man around. But when I got to be 21, I was astonished at how much the old man had learned in seven years."

To put things into context, I'm guessing most parents felt that way during our teenage years as well, but we learned better. It's up to us to attempt to reduce the negative experiences associated with that education. Nowhere is this more important than in life-threatening situations, including the encounters with drugs that most teens will certainly face.

Unfortunately, when your kids are teens, they are most likely to face one of the bigger bugaboos of young adult development–peer pressure. And with the advent of social media, your child's peer group is larger than ever, so peer pressure can be greater than any other time in history.

Mental development is most obvious in little kids, but it continues throughout childhood and young adulthood. In fact, kids experience a second "neural bloom" in the early teen years. One result is a keener sensitivity to social evaluation.[157] That means your kids care less about what you think of them; they focus instead on the opinions of those in their own age group. They feel everyone's always watching and judging them. As a result, trends and tendencies their peer group follows become more important than ever. That includes experimenting with drugs and other addictive substances.

Your best defense is to acknowledge that this increased sensitivity to peer pressure is happening, and it's perfectly natural. Even so, keep approaching your drug talks from a patient, emotionally accessible angle, listening and asking questions more than you talk. While your kids may seem to draw away from you, this occurs normally as youngsters mature and stretch their wings, so do not take it personally. Just work to be present. Adolescence provides practice for adulthood—or at least what they perceive adulthood to be. Your job is to help them get through this period with as few mistakes as possible, even if they resist you.

Your teens will probably be less receptive to your drug talks than when they were younger. They may find them boring and repetitive, so keep mixing things up. It's more important than ever that you get to know your teenager's friends and their friends' parents. Set reasonable boundaries and expectations, such as knowing where they are at all times. Insist on having a name and phone number. Call the parents to stay connected and thank them for having your son/daughter over to hang out. Make sure those parents are in alignment with your values. If the parents of your child's friends smoke weed and don't think it's a big deal, their children are 70-80% more likely to smoke pot than if their parents didn't smoke. They might even try to tempt your child into smoking if it's normalized in their home.

It's more important than ever to keep your teens apprised of new threats and support them against peer pressure. They may not want to listen; they might even push you away, but keep trying. Let them know they can call on you anytime to rescue them from a situation where one of their friends has gotten high or drunk and they feel unsafe. I remember a couple times when my children called to invoke this agreement, and I picked them up, no questions asked. They can quickly get into an unintended situation.

Now that your children are older, discuss the negative effects of drugs in more graphic detail. While details might have gone over their heads a few years ago, pointing out that today's marijuana is stronger than ever due to selective breeding will make more sense to them. THC, the active chemical in cannabis, can rise as high as 30% concentration in some strains of flower while reaching 90%+ in concentrated forms like dab or wax. Highlight not just the paranoia and psychosis effects of the hard stuff but also the IQ drops and chronic bronchitis symptoms common to long-term cannabis users. These become more evident on a day-to-day basis.

During your talks, be honest about addiction in your own family and how that may affect them. Be honest about your use, but don't glamorize it or tell stories about how you used to party.

Continue to emphasize the negative effects of drugs on the body and brain. High-potency marijuana can hospitalize a young person with one hit, especially a first-time user. They may try to use the old cliché, "Oh, *Mom*. No one has ever died from using marijuana!" But of course, that's clearly not true.

There are many indirect causes of death from using marijuana, including:

1)   It has killed people from non-stop vomiting.[158]

2)   It has killed people from house explosions.[159]

3)   It has killed people from driving while high.[160]

4)   It can also kill people from burns.[161]

5)   It can cause death by dehydration from cannabinoid hyperemesis syndrome (CHS), or cyclical vomiting, which can occur in regular users. It presents as vomiting, abdominal pain, and nausea.[162]

6)   It can cause increased suicidal ideation—clearly.[163]

Dr. Aaron Weiner, a member of Johnny's Ambassadors Scientific Advisory Board, said, "Saying that it hasn't killed anyone and thus it's okay to use is a really, really low bar. There's a lot of things that won't kill you and you still definitely shouldn't do, particularly as a teenager. Eating your shoelaces. Hugging a wild badger. Going into a room alone with R Kelly. The argument doesn't make logical sense."

Marijuana is more likely to lead to chronic psychosis[164] than any other drug studied. Sadly, about half of those who experience a marijuana-induced psychotic break will eventually develop a schizophrenia spectrum disorder.[165]

FACT: Deaths *indirectly* caused by cannabis are not rare!

So, lay down the law about marijuana use with your teens. It is your job to protect them. Make the consequences of breaking the rules clear and stick to them. If you tell them you will take away their car or phone for a month when they break your rules (and they do), *you must follow through.* If you don't, they'll see you as a pushover and won't listen to anything you say. There *must* be consequences for use of illicit substances— with zero tolerance. Don't issue a huge punishment that you can't carry out, such as "you're grounded for six months." Small beginnings can lead to huge consequences. Ask me how I know.

Some sources tell you not to express judgment when talking about drugs, especially if you discover your child has begun using. Some fear that making judgments will drive them further down the wrong path. While I agree it's easiest if your teens trust you enough to talk to you about anything, setting rules about drug use and abuse *requires* judgment.

When you make it clear that drugs are bad, you're making a judgment. When you discipline your child for experimenting or abusing drugs, you're making a judgment. If your child is abusing drugs or alcohol, there's no way you can bypass judgment. But as a parent, you must do whatever you can to protect them, so you must be *extremely* firm and take charge in getting them the help they need. Be as gentle as possible, but make no mistake, your teens must know what they've done is wrong—not necessarily from a legal or moral standpoint but because of terrible outcomes. Creating a behavior contract with your teens will let them know your expectations and spell out the consequences.

As explained throughout this book, the abuse of legal-over-21 drugs such as alcohol and marijuana can prove especially deadly to young people. These addictive substances can warp them mentally, cause psychosis, and cripple them physically. And those are just the personal costs. What they can do to others can be just as bad—from secondhand smoke to drugged driving accidents resulting in death. Don't hesitate to share parts of Johnny's story with them, too.

To summarize, use this 5E™ Process with your teens moving forward:

1) Educate — Learn all about marijuana yourself. We offer a Johnny's Ambassadors Expert Webinar Series for Parents every Friday at *https://johnnysambassadors.org/webinars*.

2) Engage — Talk to and train your children. Say, "I want to have a conversation with you about marijuana." Ask them what they know. Listen and reflect.

3) Empower — Encourage and reward good choices. Keep them off their phones as much as you can. Spend time with them and do things together. When they demonstrate the

behaviors you want, reinforce and reward them. Support their hobbies and pay for them.

4) Enforce — Protect them when poor choices are made. If your teen is under 18 and has a cannabis use disorder, send him or her to long-term residential care or recovery high school. (You can find resources on our website at *https://johnnysambassadors.org/parents.*) If having a car is enabling your teen to use marijuana and lie to you, sell the car. You're not your child's *friend*; you're your child's *parent*.

5) Escalate — If your teen verbalizes suicidality (per the C.A.R.E. Model), call the National Suicide Hotline at 800-273-8255 or 911. Your number one responsibility as a parent is to keep your child alive. I know you want your children to be loved, have a wonderful future, and be independent. All those things are wonderful, but they need to be alive for that to happen!

Can Your Child Recover?

One result of the abuse of an addictive substance like marijuana can be a substance use disorder (SUD). When it involves marijuana, it's called cannabis use disorder (CUD). All SUDs are primarily psychological ailments, though they may have physical effects if the user's brain has suffered damage from the substance abuse. A SUD can prove harder to recover from than a physical injury, and though they usually can't be seen, the scars they leave are real and often permanent.

Since the disorder was formally defined in 2013, CUD's frequency has grown along with the legalization and decriminalization of recreational marijuana use. It occurs most frequently in people under 25, a large percentage of whom are adolescents who cannot obtain marijuana legally.

SUD Recovery Methods

The brain is a delicate and complex organ. A severe SUD can damage it in ways that nothing can repair. Medical personnel and users can effectively treat SUDs, depending on the user's support system and determination to change. We had the best medical treatment available for Johnny, but he refused to participate. Because he was 18 after his first suicide attempt, he checked himself out after the first day of intensive outpatient treatment. He said he only agreed to do it to get out of the hospital, and legally, there was nothing we could do. We tried to admit him to a 12-step program, but he refused to participate. After being admitted again for psychosis, he saw a therapist twice and then refused additional treatment, only agreeing to go to his psychiatrist monthly for med refills. Then he took himself off his antipsychotics without telling anyone.

Clearly, the cooperation of the patient is critical for success. It's nearly impossible to achieve that positive change as a parent; the user must want to change. At some point, you simply can't control another human being, no matter how hard you try to help.

Most treatment programs, including 12-step programs like Alcoholics Anonymous and Narcotics Anonymous, focus on abstinence from the drug and social support from other members who have been through similar experiences. Support is crucial, whether it comes from friends, family, or 12-step comrades. As the U.S. Surgeon General's Office[166] points out, abstinence isn't enough to define recovery, "Recovery goes beyond the remission of symptoms to include a positive change in the whole person."

While emphasizing that remission from an SUD can take years and multiple rounds of treatment to fully take hold, the Surgeon General's site goes on to note that SUD recovery is more common than most people realize. At least 50% of all SUD sufferers in the U.S. have been in remission for more than a year. This applies to all users, both adolescent and adult.

The Substance Abuse and Mental Health Services Administration (SAMHSA) defines recovery from addiction as "a process of change through which individuals improve their health and wellness, live a self-directed life, and strive to reach their full potential." SAMHSA provides guidelines for living a life in recovery,[167] including these four basic dimensions for supporting such a life:

1) Maintaining one's health

2) A stable home environment

3) Maintaining purpose through meaningful daily activity (work, school, volunteering, caring for others, creative endeavors) and the means and resources to participate in society

4) Community relationships and social networks to provide support

Most recovery paths focus on total abstinence from the abused substance. One study of 119 participants[168] attributed recovery success to focusing on reasons to change, commitment to change, and conquering denial and self-deception. Several participants took advantage of some level of formal treatment while others focused purely on natural recovery based on their willpower. More than three-quarters of the participants of both types recommended treatment and use of self-help materials to sharpen their resolve. More than half also saw value in natural recovery.

Detox and Initial Recovery

The reason most recovery paths for SUDs emphasize abstinence is to purge all remaining traces of the substance from the user's system. This process can take days to weeks to six or twelve months—or longer. Dealing with the withdrawal symptoms during and following abstinence requires significant support and strength to push through them.

Again, SUDs are not purely psychological because they often cause physical brain damage. Brain scan studies[169] have revealed that some substance abusers, especially those with severe alcohol,[170] cocaine, and opioid SUDs, have suffered significant damage to both the gray and white matter in the brain. Especially affected were areas associated with the "reward system" that releases dopamine, the brain chemical that makes you feel good when you accomplish something.

Addictive substances release two to ten times the normal amount of dopamine, and they do it more often and more effectively than feel-good tasks. This short-circuits the reward system which is one reason substances are so addictive. In time, the damaged areas of the brain require more and more of the substance to work and for the user to function "normally."

Altered dopamine flow was first observed in PET brain scans of addicted individuals in a 2009 study,[171] before SUDs were formally defined. They showed the neurochemical especially low in areas associated with risk-taking and decision making. Various brain areas,[172] however, are associated with different addictive substances and activities, a factor that makes SUDs and addiction so hard to treat. Clearly, there's no single method or medication that works for everything and everyone.

Neuroplasticity

Fortunately, human brains are flexible in their response to damage and injury. Given enough time and abstinence from the substance(s) abused, they can recover most functions lost to or dulled by SUD and addiction. This ability to self-repair is called neuroplasticity.[173] It's most easily seen in adolescents and young adults whose brains are still making new connections that haven't yet been pruned away or set into stone by physical maturity.

However, older adult brains also display neuroplasticity, so any brain can somewhat heal over time. Some alcohol-related damage can heal in weeks; damage from opioids and cocaine takes more than a year for the brain to recover. Sometimes, the brain accomplishes this through the creation of new brain cells; sometimes, it just reroutes functions around the damaged areas. In addition to neuroplasticity, a 2013 study[174] indicates mindfulness training and meditation can help retrain the engrained brain pathways that normally tempt a user to relapse. Physical activity may also help.[175]

The Final Diagnosis

The milder the SUD, the easier it is to recover from. Unfortunately, the potential for relapse remains, and it's not always possible for the brain of someone with a severe SUD to fully recover. Sadly, once triggered, some mental illnesses are permanent at our present level of medical knowledge. However, users can sometimes manage them with careful and consistent use of medication.

The road is hard, and the lingering effects can be a bitter pill to swallow. However, in the final analysis, cannabis use disorder is treatable. As medical science advances and our understanding of the human brain advances with it, our options for healing from

SUDs can only grow. So, if your child has been diagnosed with an SUD such as CUD, don't despair and don't give up. Get help and stay on the lookout for new treatments and medications that can help bring them back to normalcy. Do your best, offer support, and remember you can't always control the outcome. Don't give up. Keep working to find help for your child.

EPILOGUE

The time is now. Pandora's box has been opened.

After Johnny's death, the 501(c)(3) nonprofit Johnny's Ambassadors was born. Our mission is to educate parents and teens about the dangers of today's high-THC marijuana on adolescent brain development, mental illness, and suicide. All proceeds from the sale of this book benefit Johnny's Ambassadors.

In the way of education, we will soon launch an innovative online teen curriculum to teach young people about the harmful effects of marijuana. (Get more information at *JohnnysAmbassadors.org/ curriculum.*) For parents, we offer a weekly Johnny's Ambassadors Expert Webinar Series for Parents. Past videos are on-demand at *JohnnysAmbassadors.org/recorded-webinars* and upcoming sessions at *JohnnysAmbassadors.org/webinars.*

We will be hosting an annual #StopDabbing Walk around the globe each year in September, which is Suicide Prevention Month. Register yourself or your team at *StopDabbingWalk.com.*

You may have a child, a grandchild, or a youth you work with who is affected by the dangers of marijuana. Perhaps you're concerned about a loved one's marijuana use. Maybe you have a friend whose child has struggled. It's our job as parents, grandparents, teachers, friends, law enforcement, community leaders, coalitions, counselors, and healthcare professionals— frankly, anyone with young people in their lives—to educate *ourselves* and then educate our children.

Will you please be one of Johnny's Ambassadors? Join us! Please see all the ways you can get involved at *JohnnysAmbassadors.org/join*. We are working together to save our youth from the ills of marijuana. We aim to shatter the myth that marijuana is harmless and teach people about the dangers of TODAY'S marijuana.

Please share Johnny's story with your kids of all ages. Tell them the shortened version: Johnny Stack lived in Colorado and discovered marijuana at a high school party when he was 14. He started dabbing high-THC marijuana (a very potent concentrated form), which triggered bizarre episodes of psychosis and delusional thinking (the FBI was after him, the world "knew about him," the mob had it in for him, we were "in on it," etc.). His parents disenrolled him from his current university and admitted him to a mental hospital where he was stabilized with medications. He did recover—until he used marijuana again. Eventually, even when he stopped dabbing, the psychosis did not go away, and he developed full-blown schizophrenia. Then he was put on antipsychotics to control the delusion, but he didn't like how they made him feel because he was extremely intelligent. So, he stopped taking them (a common problem with the disorder). When he died, he had given up marijuana and nicotine, he wasn't on drugs, and he wasn't depressed. But because he wouldn't take the medications he needed, the paranoid delusions told him to stop the pain, so he jumped off a building. Johnny was fiercely loved, constantly cared for, and is desperately missed. Marijuana is a sneaky, insidious beast waiting to take the life of our young ones. Do not use it, *preferably ever*, but at least until your brain is formed in your mid-to-late 20s.

Young, developing brains can't cope with the demands of today's high-THC marijuana. A teen's judgment is already impaired by puberty, as much as he or she might like to think otherwise. Teenagers' decision-making abilities aren't the best, and they may assume that something isn't dangerous to their health because it is legal. The media and pot industry make everything sound safe. But *anything* can be abused, and substances such as cannabis and alcohol have hidden dangers that adolescents may not know or understand.

A recent study[176] showed the perceived riskiness of marijuana in adolescents has been trending downward in the context of increasing legality and availability. Marijuana use varied in association with beliefs about its beneficial and harmful health properties. In other words, the less harmful our youth perceive marijuana to be, the more likely they are to use it.

As a society, we do make some efforts in schools and in the media to discourage teen substance abuse. I'm not sure, however, that we do enough to make it clear that teens *should not touch* substances that are legal for adults—not just for legal reasons, but because of biological effects that are worse for young people whose brains and bodies are still developing.

Why don't kids play with rattlesnakes? We teach them they are dangerous from an early age, and kids develop a healthy fear of rattlesnakes. The *same thing* must be done with marijuana so children have a healthy fear of what it can do to them. Mass media and the marijuana industry encourage them to use marijuana for lifestyle reasons which normalizes it in our communities, yet suicidal ideation is just one of the horrible side effects of marijuana use. Some young users are especially susceptible, and it could be someone you know and love. Remember, a neutral or non-response is effectively pro-pot. Parents, be specifically anti-pot and give a clear rebuff to your child's use of it.

I do not want any other parent to go through the hell we're going through. Please help us sound the alarm! I'm available for speaking engagements, and my travel expenses are covered through the National Marijuana Initiative Speakers Bureau. We are in a battle every day for the lives of our youth. We invite you to become one of Johnny's Ambassadors and soldier on with us. Please consider supporting our work financially at *JohnnysAmbassadors.org/donate*.

It's up to *us*—parents, grandparents, caretakers, schools, law enforcement, teachers, doctors, older siblings, youth themselves, and frankly, anyone with youth in their lives—to make a sincere, strong effort to discourage adolescent cannabis use. Even then, sometimes it's not enough. Our Johnny is lost to this poison forever.

Several people have written to me since the inception of Johnny's Ambassadors and sadly reported, "Your story is now my story." It could be your child, your grandchild, or your niece or nephew. If they are using, tell them to stop using marijuana NOW. If they aren't using, talk to them about never starting. The brain continues to form until the late 20s. That's why we must spread the word about what pot can do to kids (and to some adults, but youth are our mission). I don't want to see any other families damaged by the suicidal effects of marijuana use.

Johnny was an incredible young man hidden behind the smokescreen of marijuana, from which our legislators and society failed to protect him. What men plan for evil, God uses for His purposes. Let's spread the message for Johnny and all of our children!

ACKNOWLEDGMENTS

This is the most significant book I've ever written and the one I least wanted to write. But I promised Johnny he would do something important in the world, and I pray this book helps fulfill that promise.

Countless people have helped me through this difficult time. My greatest thanks go to my husband John, who is my rock and the center of my world. When I'm feeling fragile, he is my strength. When I'm feeling lost, he is the light in the darkness. When I'm feeling sad, he brings me joy. Through all the seasons of my life, John has given me his steadfast love, and I'm truly grateful.

I cherish my children Meagan and James, who soothe my broken heart. They were the reason I got out of bed in the morning during my darkest days. Their futures give me hope. Losing a sibling has been very difficult for them, and I admire their strength and resilience as they move through their journeys. They both sit on the board of directors for Johnny's Ambassadors and help us work to keep his spirit alive.

My gratitude goes to my extended family and close friends, who surrounded us when Johnny died. I love you all. I appreciate the support and encouragement I receive from my 5S Sisters mastermind group (I'm sworn to secrecy on why we're called the 5S Sisters): Kristin Arnold, Maribeth Kuzmeski, Marilyn Sherman, and Amy Tolbert.

There are several people in my life I simply wouldn't be able to function without: Nadine Balabanoff, the office manager of our for-profit companies; Evann Duplantier, my technology manager; and Tessa Cornelia, my personal assistant. I'm grateful for the myriad ways you support my personal and professional worlds.

My appreciation goes to the people who helped make this book a reality, including my agent, Greg Johnson of WordServe Literary Group, and my publisher, Tom Freiling of Freiling Publishing. Thank you to the reviewers who read early drafts of this book and helped make it better: Jan Typher, Sally Schindel, Cheryl Lima, Sarah Pare, Amanda Bohrer, Nancy Henderson, and Christine Miller. I'm grateful to Barbara McNichol, who has edited all of my books, and my researcher, Floyd Largent. My thanks especially go to Kevin Sabet, President and CEO of Smart Approaches to Marijuana (SAM), for writing the foreword to this book. While I've been in business for thirty years, I'm a newcomer to the nonprofit world and the marijuana industry. He trusted me enough to attach his name to our work, and I'm forever grateful for his partnership.

My extreme gratitude goes to our board of directors, who have given countless hours of their time and talent to guide Johnny's Ambassadors with their strategic wisdom: Dianna Booher, Mellanie True Hills, Robin Thompson, and Adrienne Leonard. In addition, our advisory council, consisting of leaders from our allied organizations (*www.JohnnysAmbassadors.org/ alliance*), meets with me regularly to give operational advice: Heidi Anderson-Swan with anightinjail.com; Debbie Berndt of parentmovement2-0.org; Diane Carlson of smartcolorado. org; Jacque Christmas of avoiceatthetable.org; Ben Cort of forgingnewlives.com; Kari Eckert of robbies-hope.com; Luke Niforatos of learnaboutsam.org; and Sally Schindel of mvaa.info.

A huge thanks to our major donors, whose extreme generosity launched Johnny's Ambassadors (JohnnysAmbassadors.org/ individual-ambassadors); our company sponsors, whose corporate values align with ours (JohnnysAmbassadors.org/sponsors-donors); and the hundreds of individual ambassadors, whose financial support sustains our daily operations and projects. We literally wouldn't be able to do our important work without all of you.

I'm the only staff member of Johnny's Ambassadors, so we rely on a lot of volunteers to keep our operations running smoothly. Thank you for your selfless gift of time: John Stack, Chairman and CFO; Mark Camacho and Ryan Powell, videographers; Hanna Lushchyk, website developer; Brian Walter, multimedia expert; our #StopDabbing Walk team (stopdabbingwalk.com), Steve Replin, attorney; Angie Phetteplace, accountant; Jan Typher, editor; Lisa Rue, Ph.D., curriculum designer and writer; and Jane Dvorak, public relations.

Since I'm not a clinician, I rely on our Johnny's Ambassadors Scientific Advisory Board for expert medical guidance. Thanks to Christian Thurstone, M.D., director of behavioral health at Denver Health and professor of psychiatry at the University of Colorado School of Medicine; Libby Stuyt, M.D., addiction psychiatrist at the Pueblo Community Health Center and clinical faculty member of the CU School of Medicine Department of Psychiatry; Kenneth P. Finn, M.D., who has practiced pain medicine for 24 years and is an executive board member of the American Board of Pain Medicine; Erik Messamore, M.D., an Associate Professor of Psychiatry at the NE Ohio Medical University (NEOMED) and the medical director of NEOMED's Best Practices in Schizophrenia Treatment Center; Karen Randall, M.D., an emergency medicine physician practicing in southern Colorado; Aaron Weiner, Ph.D., a practicing clinical psychologist, specializing in the treatment of individuals suffering from the consequences of drug or alcohol use or behavioral addictions; and Crystal Collier, Ph.D., LPC-S, whose areas of expertise include adolescent brain development, parent coaching, and family of origin therapy.

We're grateful to those who have written to share with us about the harms of marijuana to their children. Thank you for speaking out! You can read their stories at JohnnysAmbassadors.org/share and the stories of those who have lost children at JohnnysAmbassadors.org/memorial.

Thanks to the thousands of Johnny's Ambassadors around the world who engage in our Facebook group, participate in our events, and subscribe to our newsletter. They share our mission to educate parents and teens about the dangers of today's high-THC marijuana on adolescent brain development, mental illness, and suicide.

Finally, I thank God. The Bible tells us to rejoice always, pray constantly, and give thanks in all circumstances. Jesus continues to comfort me through this ordeal. Our Christian faith teaches that once you ask Jesus into your heart, he never departs from you, and we are saved by grace through faith. So, I know beyond a shadow of a doubt that when Johnny died, the Lord held him in His arms. Johnny is no longer tormented, and we will see him again when we leave this world to join Jesus in heaven. Even though our hearts are broken, God does give us something worth trusting in tough times–HIM. Hallelujah and Amen.

ABOUT THE AUTHOR

"Forge ahead despite your pain and give meaning to your loss."
— Laura Stack

Laura Stack is Johnny Stack's mom. In the business world, she is known by her professional moniker, The Productivity Pro® (http://www.theproductivitypro.com). She is a Hall-of-Fame Speaker and corporate spokesperson for many major brands. Laura is a bestselling author of eight books on productivity and performance topics with a large social media following. She has delivered keynote speeches and training seminars to major corporate, association, and government audiences for nearly 30 years.

On November 20, 2019, Laura had to acquire the undesired experience of knowing what it's like to lose a child. On that day, her 19-year-old son Johnny died by suicide. He suffered from delusions caused by marijuana-induced psychosis and thought the mob was after him.

That's when Laura's world took a sudden turn. She filed for and received 501(c)(3) nonprofit status for Johnny's Ambassadors, Inc. Its mission is to educate parents and teens about the dangers of today's high-THC marijuana on adolescent brain development, mental illness, and suicide. Described as a woman with unstoppable drive and unwavering purpose, Laura aims to help parents, grandparents, teachers (and all adults who have teens in their lives) by honestly and boldly sharing Johnny's story of his high-potency marijuana use, psychosis, and suicide.

Laura's platform now brings education, awareness, and a prevention curriculum to parents, organizations, healthcare professionals, community groups, and schools to raise awareness of THC use, mental illness, and suicide. By sharing Johnny's own warning about marijuana, Laura helps educate parents to talk with their children about the potential harms of today's marijuana. She is determined to start a movement to bring teen marijuana use, mental illness, and suicide into the spotlight—and get adolescents to #StopDabbing.

Laura lives with her husband John near Denver, Colorado, and has two surviving adult children, Meagan and James.

Connect with Laura Stack and Johnny's Ambassadors:

Phone: (303) 471-7401
Email: Laura@JohnnysAmbassadors.org
Website: JohnnysAmbassadors.org
Speaking Inquiries (virtual and in person): JohnnysAmbassadors.org/speaking
Twitter: @laurastack (personal) and @johnnykstack (Johnny's Ambassadors)
Facebook: Facebook.com/groups/JohnnysAmbassadors
LinkedIn: Linkedin.com/in/laurastack
YouTube: YouTube.com/JohnnysAmbassadors

AFTERWORD

On June 8, 2021, after the original publication date of this book, the Colorado legislature signed Colorado House Bill 1317 Regulating Marijuana Concentrates (http://leg.colorado.gov/bills/hb21-1317). Nearly ten years after the passage of legal recreational marijuana, the Colorado legislature recognized how high-potency marijuana can harm young people and put this important regulatory measure into place. The bill passed unanimously 35-0 in the Senate and 58-7 in the House, making it veto-proof from Governor Jared Polis. This was unheard of even a year ago.

So, early indicators are the bill is working to keep marijuana out of the hands of our youth using it as a party drug, while still allowing access by those with debilitating medical conditions. In April 2015, there were nearly 6,000 medical marijuana cards for young adults ages 18-to-20, and in August 2022, there were only 2,000!

How did this come about? In summer 2020, I was contacted by Dawn Reinfeld, a parent and activist in Boulder, CO. She came across one of my Facebook posts about Johnny and reached out to introduce herself. She wanted to run a bill to regulate THC products in Colorado and asked for my help to educate the legislators about the dangers of marijuana use in adolescents. She wanted me to tell the story of Johnny's psychosis and suicide and describe how easy it was for an 18-year-old to legally obtain a medical marijuana card and illegally sell to younger children.

Dubious but willing, John and I and several others arrived at her home on August 6, 2020, and we met in the backyard with Colorado Senate Majority Leader, Steve Fenberg, as well as Representative Judy Amabile, whose family had also been severely impacted by marijuana. We cried as we shared what happened to Johnny, and Senator Fenberg was compassionate but confused—he had no idea what dabbing was.

This began a journey of countless meetings with senators, representatives, congresspeople, and Attorney General Phil Weiser, sharing Johnny's story and his warning, "Marijuana ruined my mind and my life." Each time, I cried, as our grief was still so fresh then. It took a lot out of me emotionally, and I was unsure if anything would ever come of it. But then, incredibly, important bill sponsors signed on (Speaker Alec Garnett, Representative Yadira Caraveo, M.D., Senator Chris Hansen, and Senator Paul Lundeen, with support from Senator Kevin Priola and Representative Tim Geitner), plus twelve lobbyists from Blue Rising, Smart Colorado, Healthier Colorado, Colorado Christian University, Colorado School Nurses Association, and others. Many parents, legislators, doctors, educators, and organizations stood in support of the bill, including the Colorado Association of School Boards, Colorado Association of School Executives, and Colorado Education Association. I started to see a glimmer of hope and kept speaking out.

Originally, the bill called for a THC potency cap of 15%, and the marijuana industry sniveled so loudly, the provision was changed to fund the Colorado School of Public Health to conduct a systematic review of the scientific research related to the possible physical and mental health effects of high-potency THC concentrates on the developing brain. Their findings will inform future regulations and policy decisions at the Capitol. We will then be back with a new science-based recommendation for a THC potency cap.

The bill also:

• Tightens regulations around medical marijuana, adding new restrictions on access to potent THC products for people ages 18-20. Two physicians from different medical practices must diagnose the patient as having a debilitating or disabling medical condition after an in-person consultation. One physician must explain the risks and benefits to the patient, and one physician must provide the patient with written documentation concluding the patient might benefit from the use of medical marijuana.

• Ensures medical marijuana patients have a bonafide relationship with their doctors, so it's not as easy for people ages 18-20 to obtain cards. They must follow up with the doctor every six months to monitor their condition.

- Requires a full assessment of the patient's medical and mental health history. If the recommending physician is not the patient's primary care physician, the bill directs the recommending physician to review the records of a diagnosing physician or licensed mental health provider.
- Requires reports to be compiled from emergency room and hospital discharge data of patients with marijuana-related admissions and hospitalizations.
- Restricts daily purchase limits for concentrates like wax and shatter to 8 grams per person and 2 grams for buyers ages 18-20.
- Creates a real-time database of point-of-sale transactions, so the daily limits will now be enforced. People can no longer "loop" from dispensary to dispensary, buying over their daily limit and re-selling it.
- Requires coroners to conduct a toxicology screen on all non-natural deaths (suicide, overdose, accidental) in young people.
- Prohibits advertising directed to young people and requires marijuana advertising to include a warning regarding the risks of concentrate overconsumption.
- Directs dispensaries to provide guidance for consumers on potency and serving size.

John and I went to the Capitol several times to testify before House and Senate committees. In the second reading on the House floor, we cried as Representative Tim Geitner closed his arguments by reading my testimony to the entire assembly. I cried even harder when they rose to their feet to honor Johnny and support the bill. I then realized it was really going to happen.

This legislation is not the work of a bunch of "prohibitionists." The Colorado legislature's overwhelming approval validates the warnings we've heard from physicians, educators, parents, and our communities. It will rein in the marijuana industry, protect Colorado youth from high-potency products, and ultimately save lives.

Johnny was a victim. If this bill had been in place years ago when Johnny was entering high school, he might still be alive today. He would not have had access to the marijuana easily obtained by his friend's brother, who had a medical marijuana card. Johnny wouldn't have been able to get a card at 18 years old with no legitimate medical issues. With the new bill, the criminal "pot shop doctors" will be severely limited in their ability to sell our young people medical marijuana cards for profit.

Please understand this overhaul doesn't prevent those children who use marijuana as medicine from getting it. There are a couple hundred children in Colorado ages 17 years old and younger with medical marijuana cards who have seizures, severe autism, and other chronic medical conditions made better by marijuana components. We do not want to prevent these children from receiving help, and those currently benefiting are exempted from these new requirements when they turn 18. However, no child should have access to this toxic, mind-altering drug in the first place without a legitimate debilitating condition that warrants it. This bill simply protects the public from harm due to the overreach of the marijuana industry, just as we do with legal tobacco and opiate manufacturers. It protects children on both ends of the spectrum.

Pandora's box has been opened, and there is no turning back. If your state (or our nation) is thinking about legalization, look to the lessons Colorado learned the hard way and create similar safeguards to protect your youth. Put public health over the addiction-for-profit interests of the marijuana industry, and you'll save countless generations of youth from mental illness and suicide.

Fast forward to nearly three years after Johnny's death, November 2022, as of this writing. Johnny's Ambassadors has grown by leaps and bounds to over 10,000 around the U.S. and the world whose children and families have been harmed by marijuana use. We have over 350 Parents of Children with Cannabis-Induced Psychosis (POCCIP) right now in our private support group. John and I travel across the U.S., speaking at middle schools, high schools, universities, drug prevention conferences, parent nights, and community events (https://JohnnysAmbassadors.org/speaking). Our media has included the NYT, WSJ, PBS, and Dr. Phil (https://JohnnysAmbassadors.org/media). We know our efforts are working, as more people are sounding the alarm about high-THC products and youth psychosis, mental illness, and suicide.

My most treasured moments are having teens come up to me after talking at a school assembly, saying, "I want to thank you for sharing your son's story and this information with us today. I'm using marijuana, and after hearing you, I think I might have a problem. I'm going to get help and try to stop." There could be no greater blessing to me in the world.

I am honored to be able to keep my son's spirit alive by sharing his story. Johnny, you were right all along—marijuana did destroy your mind and your life—and you are vindicated. I will never stop sharing your warning and working to keep others from following your path. As promised, you are doing something important in this world after all.

ENDNOTES

1. Caspi, Avshalom, et al. "Moderation of the Effect of Adolescent-Onset Cannabis Use on Adult Psychosis by a Functional Polymorphism in the Catechol-O-Methyltransferase Gene: Longitudinal Evidence of a Gene X Environment Interaction." *Biological Psychiatry*, vol. 57, no. 10, 22 Mar. 2005, pp. 1117–1127., DOI: https://doi.org/10.1016/j.biopsych.2005.01.026.

2. National Institute on Drug Abuse. *Marijuana Potency*. 8 July 2020, www.drugabuse.gov/drug-topics/marijuana/marijuana-potency.

3. Stuyt, Elizabeth. "The Problem with the Current High Potency THC Marijuana from the Perspective of an Addiction Psychiatrist." Missouri Medicine, vol. 115,6 (2018): 482-486.

4. Gillespie, Claire. "'Dabbing' Pot is The New Dangerous Trend Among Teens—Here's What to Know." Health.com, 18 Feb. 2020, www.health.com/condition/smoking/dangers-of-dabbing-pot.

5. Gogtay, Nitin, et al. "Dynamic mapping of human cortical development during childhood through early adulthood." *Proceedings of the National Academy of Sciences of the United States of America,* vol. 101,21 (2004): 8174-9. DOI: 10.1073/pnas.0402680101.

6. NIDA. "What are marijuana's long-term effects on the brain?" *National Institute on Drug Abuse*, 8 Apr. 2020, https://www.drugabuse.gov/publications/research-reports/marijuana/what-are-marijuanas-long-term-effects-brain. Accessed 13 Mar. 2021.

7. Di Forti, Marta, et al. "Daily use, especially of high-potency cannabis, drives the earlier onset of psychosis in cannabis users." *Schizophrenia bulletin* vol. 40,6 (2014): 1509-17. DOI: 10.1093/schbul/sbt181.

8. Price, Ceri, et al. "Cannabis and suicide: longitudinal study." *The British Journal of Psychiatry: the Journal of Mental Science,* vol. 195,6 (2009): 492-7. DOI: 10.1192/bjp.bp.109.065227.

9. Lopez-Quintero, Catalina et al. "Probability and predictors of transition from first use to dependence on nicotine, alcohol, cannabis, and cocaine: results of the National Epidemiologic Survey on Alcohol and Related Conditions (NESARC)." *Drug and Alcohol Dependence,* vol. 115,1-2 (2011): 120-30. DOI: 10.1016/j.drugalcdep.2010.11.004.

10. Hlavinka, Elizabeth. "Meta-Analysis: Even One THC Hit Carries Risk for Inducing Psychosis." *Medical News and Free CME Online,* MedpageToday, 17 Mar. 2020, ww.medpagetoday.com/psychiatry/generalpsychiatry/85472.

11. https://georgespicka.weebly.com/marijuana-links.html.

12. Thompson, Dennis. "Study: Today's Stronger Pot Is More Addictive." *WebMD,* 17 Dec. 2018, www.webmd.com/mental-health/addiction/news/20181217/study-todays-stronger-pot-is-more-addictive.

13. Volkow, Nora, et al. "Adverse Health Effects of Marijuana Use." *New England Journal of Medicine,* vol. 370, no. 23, 11 Apr. 2016, pp. 2219–2227., DOI: 10.1056/NEJMra1402309.

14. Meier, Madeline H., et al. "Persistent Cannabis Users Show Neuropsychological Decline from Childhood to Midlife." *PNAS,* National Academy of Sciences, 2 Oct. 2012, www.pnas.org/content/109/40/E2657.

15. Barrington-Trimis, Jessica L., et al. "Risk of Persistence and Progression of Use of 5 Cannabis Products After Experimentation Among Adolescents." *JAMA Network Open,* American Medical Association, 3 Jan. 2020, www.ncbi.nlm.nih.gov/pmc/articles/PMC6991277/.

16. Fiellin, Lynn E., et al. "Prior Use of Alcohol, Cigarettes, and Marijuana and Subsequent Abuse of Prescription Opioids in Young Adults." *Journal of Adolescent Health,* vol. 52, no. 2, Feb. 2013, pp. 158–163., DOI: 10.1016/j.jadohealth.2012.06.010.

17. Nourbakhsh, Mahra, et al. "Cannabinoid Hyperemesis Syndrome: Reports of Fatal Cases." *Journal of Forensic Sciences* vol. 64,1 (2019): 270-274. DOI: 10.1111/1556-4029.13819.

18. Lynskey, M., and W. Hall. "The effects of adolescent cannabis use on educational attainment: a review." *Addiction (Abingdon, England),* vol. 95,11 (2000): 1621-30. DOI: 10.1046/j.1360-0443.2000.951116213.x.

19. Marconi, Arianna, et al. "Meta-analysis of the Association Between the Level of Cannabis Use and Risk of Psychosis." *Schizophrenia Bulletin,* vol. 42,5 (2016): 1262-9. DOI: 10.1093/schbul/sbw003.

20. Gundersen, Tina Djernis, et al. "Association Between Use of Marijuana and Male Reproductive Hormones and Semen Quality: A Study Among 1,215

Healthy Young Men." *American Journal of Epidemiology,* vol. 182,6 (2015): 473-81. DOI: 10.1093/aje/kwv135.

21. University College London. "Cannabis reduces short-term motivation to work for money: Smoking the equivalent of a single 'spliff' of cannabis makes people less willing to work for money while 'high'." ScienceDaily. ScienceDaily, 1 September 2016, www.sciencedaily.com/releases/2016/09/160901211303.htm.

22. Freeman, Daniel, et al. "How Cannabis Causes Paranoia: Using the Intravenous Administration of Δ 9 -Tetrahydrocannabinol (THC) to Identify Key Cognitive Mechanisms Leading to Paranoia." *OUP Academic*, Oxford University Press, 16 July 2014, cademic.oup.com/schizophreniabulletin/article/41/2/391/2526091.

23. NIDA. "What are marijuana's effects on lung health?" *National Institute on Drug Abuse*, 8 Apr. 2020, https://www.drugabuse.gov/publications/research-reports/marijuana/what-are-marijuanas-effects-lung-health. Accessed 13 Mar. 2021.

24. Compton, Richard. "Marijuana-Impaired Driving A Report to Congress." *National Highway Traffic Safety Administration*, July 2017, www.nhtsa.gov/sites/nhtsa.dot.gov/files/documents/812440-marijuana-impaired-driving-report-to-congress.pdf.

25. Bonnet, Udo, and Ulrich W. Preuss. "The cannabis withdrawal syndrome: current insights." *Substance Abuse and Rehabilitation* vol. 8 9-37. 27 Apr. 2017, DOI: 10.2147/SAR.S109576.

26. Peter Grinspoon, MD. "If Cannabis Becomes a Problem: How to Manage Withdrawal." *Harvard Health Blog*, 26 May 2020, www.health.harvard.edu/blog/if-cannabis-becomes-a-problem-how-to-manage-withdrawal-2020052619922.

27. Anees Bahji, MD. "Cannabis Withdrawal Symptoms in People with Regular or Dependent Cannabinoid Use." *JAMA Network Open*, JAMA Network, 9 Apr. 2020, jamanetwork.com/journals/jamanetworkopen/fullarticle/2764234.

28. Leung, Janni, et al. "What Is the Prevalence and Risk of Cannabis Use Disorders among People Who Use Cannabis? A Systematic Review and Meta-Analysis." *Addictive Behaviors*, Pergamon, 20 May 2020, www.sciencedirect.com/science/article/abs/pii/S0306460320306092.

29. Peter Grinspoon, MD. "If Cannabis Becomes a Problem: How to Manage Withdrawal." *Harvard Health Blog*, 26 May 2020, www.health.harvard.

edu/blog/if-cannabis-becomes-a-problem-how-to-manage-withdraw-al-2020052619922.

30. "Vaping and Marijuana: What You Need to Know." *Partnership to End Addiction*, May 2020, drugfree.org/article/vaping-and-marijuana-what-you-need-to-know/.

31. Conkiln, Mark. "Why Does Marijuana Cause Red Eyes & What to Do About It." *THC Physicians*, 14 Dec. 2020, thcphysicians.com/does-marijua-na-cause-red-eyes/.

32. "Is It Possible to 'Overdose' or Have a 'Bad Reaction' to Marijuana?" *Centers for Disease Control and Prevention*, 7 Mar. 2018, www.cdc.gov/marijua-na/faqs/overdose-bad-reaction.html.

33. Galli, Jonathan A., et al. "Cannabinoid hyperemesis syndrome." *Current Drug Abuse Reviews* vol. 4,4 (2011): 241-9. DOI: 10.2174/1874473711104040241.

34. "How to Tell Your Child Is Smoking Weed: Sober College." *Become a Drug & Alcohol Certified Addictions Counselor | Sober College*, 16 Dec. 2019, so-bercollege.com/addiction-blog/signs-your-child-is-smoking-pot/.

35. Sison, Gerardo. "3 Signs Your Teen May Be Using Marijuana: Weed Addic-tion & Treatment." *American Addiction Centers*, 14 Oct. 2019, americanad-dictioncenters.org/marijuana-rehab/signs-of-marijuana-use-in-teens.

36. Santos-Longhurst, Adrienne. "Blunts, Spliffs, and Joints: What to Know Before You Roll Up." *Healthline.com*, 21 Oct. 2019, www.healthline.com/health/what-is-a-blunt.

37. Driscoll Jorgensen, Elizabeth. "Dabs, Wax, Vaping Weed, Edibles and the Real Impact of High Potency THC Products: What Parents Need to Know." *Resources To Recover*, 15 Oct. 2019, www.rtor.org/2019/09/16/dabs-wax-va-ping-weed-edibles-what-parents-need-to-know/?fbclid=IwAR1FfZqV2R6d-FLEvlFfAJGvdGtuaBwrYJQpB1D3Whtc4BkobMSWWnZ3EnTI.

38. "How to Tell Your Child Is Smoking Weed: Sober College." *Become a Drug & Alcohol Certified Addictions Counselor | Sober College*, 16 Dec. 2019, so-bercollege.com/addiction-blog/signs-your-child-is-smoking-pot/.

39. Volkow, Nora, et al. "Adverse Health Effects of Marijuana Use." *New En-gland Journal of Medicine*, vol. 370, no. 23, 11 Apr. 2016, pp. 2219–2227., DOI: 10.1056/NEJMra1402309.

40. Agrawal, Arpana, et al. "Major depressive disorder, suicidal thoughts and behaviours, and cannabis involvement in discordant twins: a retrospec-tive cohort study." *The Lancet. Psychiatry* vol. 4,9 (2017): 706-714. DOI: 10.1016/S2215-0366(17)30280-8.

41. Gates, Dr. Peter. "Does Cannabis Cause Mental Illness?" *NDARC*, https://ndarc.med.unsw.edu.au/blog/does-Cannabis-cause-mental-illness.

42. Budney, Alan J., et al. "The time course and significance of cannabis withdrawal." *Journal of Abnormal Psychology*, vol. 112,3 (2003): 393-402. DOI: 10.1037/0021-843x.112.3.393.

43. Hayatbakhsh, Mohammad R., et al. "Cannabis and anxiety and depression in young adults: a large prospective study." *Journal of the American Academy of Child and Adolescent Psychiatry*, vol. 46,3 (2007): 408-417. DOI: 10.1097/chi.0b013e31802dc54d.

44. Thomas, Huw. "A Community Survey of Adverse Effects of Cannabis Use." *Science Direct*, vol. 42, no. 3, Nov. 1996, pp. 201–207., DOI: https://doi.org/10.1016/S0376-8716(96)01277-X.

45. Andreasson, Sven, et al. "CANNABIS AND SCHIZOPHRENIA A Longitudinal Study of Swedish Conscripts," vol. 330, no. 8574, 26 Dec. 1987, pp. 1483–1486., DOI: https://doi.org/10.1016/S0140-6736(87)92620-1.

46. Price, Ceri, et al. "Cannabis and suicide: longitudinal study." *The British Journal of Psychiatry: the Journal of Mental Science*, vol. 195,6 (2009): 492-7. DOI: 10.1192/bjp.bp.109.065227.

47. www.samhsa.gov/data/sites/default/files/NSDUH-DetTabs2014/NSDUH-DetTabs2014.pdf.

48. Tice, Peter. "RESULTS FROM THE 2014 NATIONAL SURVEY ON DRUG USE AND HEALTH: DETAILED TABLES." *www.samhsa.gov*, 10 Sept. 2015, pp. 1–2404.

49. "Results from the 2018 National Survey on Drug Use and Health: Detailed Tables." *www.samhsa.gov*, 2019, www.samhsa.gov/data/sites/default/files/cbhsq-reports/NSDUHDetailedTabs2018R2/NSDUHDetTabsSect1pe2018.htm.

50. Gold, Mark S., et al. "Marijuana Addictive Disorders: DSM-5 Substance-Related Disorders." *OMICS International*, OMICS International, 16 Jan. 2017, www.omicsonline.org/open-access/marijuana-addictive-disorders-and-dsm5-substancerelated-disorders-2155-6105-S11-013.php?aid=84734.

51. Gold, Mark S., et al. "Marijuana Addictive Disorders: DSM-5 Substance-Related Disorders." *OMICS International*, OMICS International, 16 Jan. 2017, www.omicsonline.org/open-access/marijuana-addictive-disorders-and-dsm5-substancerelated-disorders-2155-6105-S11-013.php?aid=84734.

52. Leung, Janni, et al. "What Is the Prevalence and Risk of Cannabis Use Disorders among People Who Use Cannabis? A Systematic Review and Me-

ta-Analysis." *Addictive Behaviors*, Pergamon, 20 May 2020, www.sciencedi-rect.com/science/article/abs/pii/S0306460320306092?via%3Dihub.

53. https://johnnysambassadors.org/wp-content/uploads/2020/09/Key-Sub-stance-Use.pdf.

54. "Self-Help for Sobriety Without Relapse." *Oxford House*, www.oxfordhouse.org/userfiles/file/.

55. Williams, Arthur Robin. "Cannabis as a Gateway Drug for Opioid Use Disorder." *The Journal of Law, Medicine & Ethics: a Journal of the American Society of Law, Medicine & Ethics*, vol. 48,2 (2020): 268-274. DOI: 10.1177/1073110520935338.

56. Volkow, Nora, et al. "Adverse Health Effects of Marijuana Use." *New England Journal of Medicine*, vol. 370, no. 23, 11 Apr. 2016, pp. 2219–2227., DOI: 10.1056/NEJMra1402309.

57. Gaffuri, Anne-Lise, et al. "Type-1 cannabinoid receptor signaling in neuronal development." *Pharmacology*, vol. 90,1-2 (2012): 19-39. DOI: 10.1159/000339075.

58. Silins, Edmund, et al. "Young Adult Sequelae of Adolescent Cannabis Use: an Integrative Analysis." *The Lancet*, vol. 1, no. 4, Sept. 2014, pp. 286–293., DOI: https://doi.org/10.1016/S2215-0366(14)70307-4.

59. "The Impact of Adolescent Cannabis Use, Mood Disorder and Lack of Education on Attempted Suicide in Young Adulthood." *World Psychiatry*, vol. 13, no. 3, Oct. 2014, pp. 322–323., DOI: 10.1002/wps.20170.

60. Sellers, Christina, et al. "Alcohol and Marijuana Use as Daily Predictors of Suicide Ideation and Attempts among Adolescents Prior to Psychiatric Hospitalization." *Elsevier*, vol. 273, Mar. 2019, pp. 672–677., DOI: https://doi.org/10.1016/j.psychres.2019.02.006.

61. *Workbook: CoVDRS_12.1.17*, Colorado Center for Health and Environmental Data, cohealthviz.dphe.state.co.us/t/HSEBPublic/views/Co-VDRS_12_1_17/Story1?%3Aembed=y&%3AshowAppBanner=false&%3A-showShareOptions=true&%3Adisplay_count=no&%3AshowVizHome=no#.

62. Volkow, Nora, et al. "Adverse Health Effects of Marijuana Use." *New England Journal of Medicine*, vol. 370, no. 23, 11 Apr. 2016, pp. 2219–2227., DOI: 10.1056/NEJMra1402309.

63. Price, Ceri, et al. "Cannabis and suicide: longitudinal study." *The British Journal of Psychiatry: the Journal of Mental Science*, vol. 195,6 (2009): 492-7. DOI: 10.1192/bjp.bp.109.065227.

64. https://johnnysambassadors.org/wp-content/uploads/2020/09/Apply-ing-the-Bradford-Hill-criteria-to-the-marijuana-suicide-question.pdf.

65. Colizzi, Marco, and Robin Murray. "Cannabis and Psychosis: What Do We Know and What Should We Do?" *The British Journal of Psychiatry*, vol. 212, no. 4, 2018, pp. 195–196., DOI: 10.1192/bjp.2018.1.

66. Henquet, Cécile, et al. "Prospective Cohort Study of Cannabis Use, Predis-position for Psychosis, and Psychotic Symptoms in Young People." *Ncbi. nlm.nih.gov*, pp. 1–4., www.ncbi.nlm.nih.gov/pmc/articles/PMC539839/pdf/bmj33000011.pdf.

67. Marconi, Arianna, et al. "Meta analysis of the Association Between the Level of Cannabis Use and Risk of Psychosis." *Schizophrenia Bulletin,* vol. 42,5 (2016): 1262-9. DOI: 10.1093/schbul/sbw003.

68. Di Forti, Marta, et al. "Proportion of Patients in South London with First-Episode Psychosis Attributable to Use of High Potency Cannabis: a Case-Control Study." *The Lancet*, vol. 2, no. 3, 1 Mar. 2015, pp. 233–238., DOI: https://doi.org/10.1016/S2215-0366(14)00117-5.

69. Konings, M., et al. "Early Exposure to Cannabis and Risk for Psychosis in Young Adolescents in Trinidad." *Acta Psychiatrica Scandinavica*, vol. 118, no. 3, 2008, pp. 209–213., DOI: 10.1111/j.1600-0447.2008.01202.x.

70. https://johnnysambassadors.org/johnny-stacks-story/.

71. Bonnet, Udo, and Ulrich W. Preuss. "The cannabis withdrawal syndrome: current insights." *Substance Abuse and Rehabilitation,* vol. 8 9-37. 27 Apr. 2017, DOI: 10.2147/SAR.S109576.

72. "Schizophrenia and Suicide: Risk Factors and Suicide Prevention." *WebMD*, www.webmd.com/schizophrenia/schizophrenia-and-suicide#1.

73. Bonnet, Udo, and Ulrich W. Preuss. "The cannabis withdrawal syndrome: current insights." *Substance Abuse and Rehabilitation,* vol. 8 9-37. 27 Apr. 2017, DOI: 10.2147/SAR.S109576.

74. Oberbarnscheidt, Thersilla, and Norman Miller. "The Impact of Cannabi-diol on Psychiatric and Medical Conditions," vol. 12, no. 7, 25 June 2020, DOI: 10.14740/jocmr4159.

75. https://www.facebook.com/laurastack/posts/10157239177009472.

76. http://www.theproductivitypro.com/.

77. https://www.facebook.com/laurastack/posts/10157274878294472.

78. https://johnnysambassadors.org/johnny-stacks-story/.

79. "420 (Cannabis Culture)." *Wikipedia*, Wikimedia Foundation, 4 Feb. 2021, en.wikipedia.org/wiki/420_(cannabis_culture).

80. Volkow, Nora, et al. "Adverse Health Effects of Marijuana Use." *New England Journal of Medicine*, vol. 370, no. 23, 11 Apr. 2016, pp. 2219–2227., DOI: 10.1056/NEJMra1402309.

81. Denny, Regina. "My Experience of Cannabinoid Hyperemesis Syndrome (CHS)." *Medical News Today*, MediLexicon International, 19 Sept. 2019, www.medicalnewstoday.com/articles/326357.

82. Gold, Mark S., et al. "Marijuana Addictive Disorders: DSM-5 Substance-Related Disorders." *OMICS International*, OMICS International, 16 Jan. 2017, www.omicsonline.org/open-access/marijuana-addictive-disorders-and-dsm5-substancerelated-disorders-2155-6105-S11-013.php?aid=84734.

83. Gold, Mark S., et al. "Marijuana Addictive Disorders: DSM-5 Substance-Related Disorders." *OMICS International*, OMICS International, 16 Jan. 2017, www.omicsonline.org/open-access/marijuana-addictive-disorders-and-dsm5-substancerelated-disorders-2155-6105-S11-013.php?aid=84734.

84. Gold, Mark S., et al. "Marijuana Addictive Disorders: DSM-5 Substance-Related Disorders." *OMICS International*, OMICS International, 16 Jan. 2017, www.omicsonline.org/open-access/marijuana-addictive-disorders-and-dsm5-substancerelated-disorders-2155-6105-S11-013.php?aid=84734.

85. Gold, Mark S., et al. "Marijuana Addictive Disorders: DSM-5 Substance-Related Disorders." *OMICS International*, OMICS International, 16 Jan. 2017, www.omicsonline.org/open-access/marijuana-addictive-disorders-and-dsm5-substancerelated-disorders-2155-6105-S11-013.php?aid=84734.

86. "Outbreak of Lung Injury Associated with the Use of E-Cigarette, or Vaping, Products." *Centers for Disease Control and Prevention*, 27 Nov. 2020, www.cdc.gov/tobacco/basic_information/e-cigarettes/severe-lung-disease.html?fbclid=IwAR0Lk9IpH9OMaP_2dvwO7UqKlUJklslyhchhaPTeoTYtYLEf34p4pTs5q6M.

87. Rocky Mountain High Intensity Drug Trafficking Area program. "The Legalization of Marijuana in Colorado: The Impact: Volume 6, September 2019." *Missouri Medicine,* vol. 116,6 (2019): 450.

88. Cass, D. K., et al. "CB1 cannabinoid receptor stimulation during adolescence impairs the maturation of GABA function in the adult rat prefron-

tal cortex." *Molecular Psychiatry,* vol. 19,5 (2014): 536-43. DOI: 10.1038/mp.2014.14.

89. Gold, Mark S., et al. "Marijuana Addictive Disorders: DSM-5 Substance-Related Disorders." *OMICS International,* OMICS International, 16 Jan. 2017, www.omicsonline.org/open-access/marijuana-addictive-disorders-and-dsm5-substancerelated-disorders-2155-6105-S11-013.php?aid=84734.

90. Gaffuri, Anne-Lise, et al. "Type-1 cannabinoid receptor signaling in neuronal development." *Pharmacology* vol. 90,1-2 (2012): 19-39. DOI: 10.1159/000339075.

91. Gates, Dr. Peter. "Does Cannabis Cause Mental Illness?" *NDARC,* ndarc. med.unsw.edu.au/blog/does-Cannabis-cause-mental-illness?fbclid=IwAR2l-BONOxUvMnSeaFOu9S6Oibfnuk0azS7usCN5WOE5wTE1xa24w_zddvBM.

92. Budney, Alan J., et al. "The time course and significance of cannabis withdrawal." *Journal of Abnormal Psychology,* vol. 112,3 (2003): 393-402. DOI: 10.1037/0021-843x.112.3.393.

93. Volkow, Nora, et al. "Adverse Health Effects of Marijuana Use." *New England Journal of Medicine,* vol. 370, no. 23, 11 Apr. 2016, pp. 2219–2227., DOI: 10.1056/NEJMra1402309.

94. Volkow, Nora, et al. "Adverse Health Effects of Marijuana Use." *New England Journal of Medicine,* vol. 370, no. 23, 11 Apr. 2016, pp. 2219–2227., DOI: 10.1056/NEJMra1402309.

95. Thomas, Huw. "A Community Survey of Adverse Effects of Cannabis Use." *Science Direct,* vol. 42, no. 3, Nov. 1996, pp. 201–207., DOI: https://doi.org/10.1016/S0376-8716(96)01277-X.

96. Saha, Sukanta, et al. "A systematic review of the prevalence of schizophrenia." *PLoS Medicine,* vol. 2,5 (2005): e141. DOI: 10.1371/journal.pmed.0020141.

97. https://johnnysambassadors.org/wp-content/uploads/2020/09/Applying-the-Bradford-Hill-criteria-to-the-marijuana-suicide-question.pdf?fbclid=IwAR3EK4KAU6ajhOMBhgQqYwPtkegiYfq71ufdyc0IUi6eFlasvtQjxGDTcY0.

98. Hall, Wayne, et al. "The Effects of Cannabis Use on the Development of Adolescents and Young Adults," vol. 2, Dec. 2020, pp. 461–483., DOI: https://doi.org/10.1146/annurev-devpsych-040320-084904.

99. Brody, Jane. "Mental Ills Linked to Marijuana." *New York Times,* 19 Apr. 1971, p. 24.

100. Wilson, Jack, et al. "Effects of increasing cannabis potency on adolescent health." *The Lancet. Child & Adolescent Health,* vol. 3,2 (2019): 121-128. DOI: 10.1016/S2352-4642(18)30342-0.

101. Saha, Sukanta, et al. "A systematic review of the prevalence of schizophrenia." *PLoS Medicine,* vol. 2,5 (2005): e141. DOI: 10.1371/journal. pmed.0020141.

102. Cass, D. K., et al. "CB1 cannabinoid receptor stimulation during adolescence impairs the maturation of GABA function in the adult rat prefrontal cortex." *Molecular Psychiatry,* vol. 19,5 (2014): 536-43. DOI: 10.1038/ mp.2014.14.

103. Renard, Justine, et al. "Effects of Adolescent THC Exposure on the Prefrontal GABAergic System: Implications for Schizophrenia-Related Psychopathology." *Frontiers in Psychiatry,* vol. 9, 2 July 2018, p. 281., DOI: 10.3389/fpsyt.2018.00281.

104. "UVM Homepage." *University of Vermont,* www.uvm.edu/.

105. "Medical Xpress - Medical Research Advances and Health News." *Gray Matter Volume News and Latest Updates,* medicalxpress.com/tags/ gray+matter+volume/.

106. "Medical Xpress - Medical Research Advances and Health News." *Brain News and Latest Updates,* medicalxpress.com/tags/brain/.

107. Shen, Helen. "News Feature: Cannabis and the Adolescent Brain." *Proceedings of the National Academy of Sciences,* vol. 117, no. 1, 7 Jan. 2020, pp. 7–11., DOI: 10.1073/pnas.1920325116.

108. "FDA and Cannabis: Research and Drug Approval Process." *U.S. Food and Drug Administration,* FDA, 1 Oct. 2020, www.fda.gov/news-events/public-health-focus/fda-and-cannabis-research-and-drug-approval-process.

109. Bowen, Lynneice L., and Aimee L. McRae-Clark. "Therapeutic Benefit of Smoked Cannabis in Randomized Placebo-Controlled Studies." *Pharmacotherapy,* vol. 38,1 (2018): 80-85. DOI: 10.1002/phar.2064.

110. Mack A., Joy J. Marijuana as Medicine? The Science Beyond the Controversy. Washington (DC): National Academies Press (US); 2000. 4, MARIJUANA AND PAIN. Available from: https://www.ncbi.nlm.nih.gov/books/ NBK224384/.

111. Bowen, Lynneice L., and Aimee L. McRae-Clark. "Therapeutic Benefit of Smoked Cannabis in Randomized Placebo-Controlled Studies." *Pharmacotherapy,* vol. 38,1 (2018): 80-85. DOI: 10.1002/phar.2064

112. Mack A., Joy J. Marijuana as Medicine? The Science Beyond the Controversy. Washington (DC): National Academies Press (US); 2000. 4, MARIJUANA AND PAIN. Available from: https://www.ncbi.nlm.nih.gov/books/NBK224384/.

113. Tomida, I., et al. "Cannabinoids and glaucoma." *The British Journal of Ophthalmology*, vol. 88,5 (2004): 708-13. DOI: 10.1136/bjo.2003.032250.

114. "American Academy of Ophthalmology Reiterates Position That Marijuana Is Not Proven Treatment for Glaucoma." *American Academy of Ophthalmology*, 27 June 2014, www.aao.org/newsroom/news-releases/detail/american-academy-of-ophthalmology-reiterates-posit.

115. Mack A., Joy J. Marijuana as Medicine? The Science Beyond the Controversy. Washington (DC): National Academies Press (US); 2000. 9, MARIJUANA AND GLAUCOMA. Available from: https://www.ncbi.nlm.nih.gov/books/NBK224386/.

116. "Dr. Phil & Oz Test the CBD Oil That Used Them in Fake Ads." *The Dr. Oz Show*, 17 Feb. 2021, www.doctoroz.com/episode-playlist-february-17-2021/dr-phil-oz-test-the-cbd-oil-that-used-them-in-fake-ads.

117. "Find Medical Marijuana Doctors Near You." *Marijuana Doctors*, www.marijuanadoctors.com/medical-marijuana-doctors/.

118. "What Is the Average Cost of a Marijuana Examination?" *Marijuana Doctors*, 4 Jan. 2020, www.marijuanadoctors.com/blog/cost-of-marijuana-examination/.

119. "How Much Does It Cost to Obtain an Ohio Medical Marijuana Card?" *Medical Marijuana Physicians of Ohio, LLC*, medicalmarijuanaphysiciansofohio.com/costs-and-fees/.

120. "Medical Marijuana Certification Services & Pricing at All Greens Clinic in Sun City, AZ." *All Greens Clinic*, 22 Feb. 2021, www.allgreensclinic.org/medical-marijuana-card-pricing-arizona/.

121. Sherrard, Melissa. "How Much 'Weed' Cards Cost in Every State." *Civilized*, www.civilized.life/articles/how-much-weed-cards-cost-in-every-state/.

122. http://www.johnnysambassadors.org/research.

123. Volkow, Nora D., et al. "Adverse health effects of marijuana use." *The New England Journal of Medicine*, vol. 370,23 (2014): 2219-27. DOI: 10.1056/NEJMra1402309.

124. Gaffuri, Anne-Lise, et al. "Type-1 cannabinoid receptor signaling in neuronal development." *Pharmacology*, vol. 90,1-2 (2012): 19-39. DOI: 10.1159/000339075.

125. Bergland, Christopher. "Does Long-Term Cannabis Use Stifle Motivation?" *Psychology Today*, Sussex Publishers, 2 July 2013, www.psychologytoday. com/us/blog/the-athletes-way/201307/does-long-term-cannabis-use-sti-fle-motivation.

126. Reuters. "Study: Teens Smoke Pot to Cope With Stress, Health Problems." *Fox News*, FOX News Network, 25 Mar. 2015, www.foxnews.com/story/ study-teens-smoke-pot-to-cope-with-stress-health-problems.

127. Bottorff, Joan L., et al. "Relief-oriented use of marijuana by teens." *Substance Abuse Treatment, Prevention, and Policy*, vol. 4 7. 23 Apr. 2009, DOI: 10.1186/1747-597X-4-7.

128. Grinspoon, Peter. "Medical Marijuana." *Harvard Health Blog*, 10 Apr. 2020, www.health.harvard.edu/blog/medical-marijuana-2018011513085.

129. Silins, Edmund, et al. "Young Adult Sequelae of Adolescent Cannabis Use: an Integrative Analysis." *The Lancet*, vol. 1, no. 4, Sept. 2014, pp. 286–293., DOI: https://doi.org/10.1016/S2215-0366(14)70307-4.

130. Agrawal, Arpana, et al. "Major depressive disorder, suicidal thoughts and behaviours, and cannabis involvement in discordant twins: a retrospective cohort study." *The Lancet. Psychiatry*, vol. 4,9 (2017): 706-714. DOI: 10.1016/S2215-0366(17)30280-8.

131. Budney, Alan J., et al. "The time course and significance of cannabis withdrawal." *Journal of Abnormal Psychology*, vol. 112,3 (2003): 393-402. DOI: 10.1037/0021-843x.112.3.393.

132. Hayatbakhsh, Mohammad R., et al. "Cannabis and anxiety and depression in young adults: a large prospective study." *Journal of the American Academy of Child and Adolescent Psychiatry*, vol. 46,3 (2007): 408-417. DOI: 10.1097/chi.0b013e31802dc54d.

133. Morrison, Paul D., et al. "Disruption of Frontal Theta Coherence by Δ9-Tetrahydrocannabinol Is Associated with Positive Psychotic Symptoms." *Neuropsychopharmacology*, vol. 36, no. 4, 8 Dec. 2010, pp. 827–836., DOI: 10.1038/npp.2010.222.

134. Di Forti, Marta, et al. "The Contribution of Cannabis Use to Variation in the Incidence of Psychotic Disorder across Europe (EU-GEI): a Multicentre Case-Control Study." *The Lancet Psychiatry*, vol. 6, no. 5, 19 Mar. 2019, pp. 427–436., DOI: 10.1016/s2215-0366(19)30048-3.

135. Messamore, Erik. "DOES MARIJUANA CAUSE SCHIZOPHRENIA?" *Erikmessamore.com*, 31 Jan. 2021, erikmessamore.com/does-marijua-na-cause-schizophrenia/?fbclid=IwAR1OjynnnZfwiuysXOkHu6Ul_gk7vYxP_Vn-DhOvsnuizRDF3lkesZlCmp4.

136. Colizzi, Marco, and Robin Murray. "Cannabis and psychosis: what do we know and what should we do?." *The British Journal of Psychiatry: the Journal of Mental Science,* vol. 212,4 (2018): 195-196. DOI: 10.1192/bjp.2018.1.

137. Grewal, Ruby S., and Tony P. George. "8 Distinguishing Features of Primary Psychosis Versus Cannabis-Induced Psychosis." *Psychiatric Times,* 4 Aug. 2017, www.psychiatrictimes.com/view/8-distinguishing-features-primary-psychosis-versus-cannabis-induced-psychosis.

138. Sund, Reijo, et al. "Substance-Induced Psychoses Converting Into Schizophrenia: A Register-Based Study of 18,478 Finnish Inpatient Cases." *Psychiatrist.com,* 17 Apr. 2012, www.psychiatrist.com/jcp/schizophrenia/substance-use-disorders/substance-induced-psychoses-converting-schizophrenia/.

139. Starzer, Marie Stefanie Kejser, et al. "Rates and Predictors of Conversion to Schizophrenia or Bipolar Disorder Following Substance-Induced Psychosis." *The American Journal of Psychiatry,* vol. 175,4 (2018): 343-350. DOI: 10.1176/appi.ajp.2017.17020223.

140. King, Daniel J., et al. "A Review of Abnormalities in the Perception of Visual Illusions in Schizophrenia." *Psychonomic Bulletin & Review,* vol. 24, no. 3, 11 Oct. 2016, pp. 734–751., DOI: 10.3758/s13423-016-1168-5.

141. Vadhan, Nehal P., et al. "Acute effects of smoked marijuana in marijuana smokers at clinical high-risk for psychosis: A preliminary study." *Psychiatry Research,* vol. 257 (2017): 372-374. DOI: 10.1016/j.psychres.2017.07.070.

142. Henquet, Cécile, et al. "Psychosis Reactivity to Cannabis Use in Daily Life: an Experience Sampling Study." *British Journal of Psychiatry,* vol. 196, no. 6, 2010, pp. 447–453., DOI: 10.1192/bjp.bp.109.072249.

143. "Youth Risk Behavior Surveillance System (YRBSS)." *Centers for Disease Control and Prevention,* 27 Oct. 2020, www.cdc.gov/healthyyouth/data/yrbs/index.htm.

144. "United States, High School Youth Risk Behavior Survey, 2017." *Centers for Disease Control and Prevention,* 2018, nccd.cdc.gov/Youthonline/App/Results.aspx?TT=A&OUT=0&SID=HS&QID=QQ&LID=XX-&YID=2017&LID2=&YID2=&COL=S&ROW1=N&ROW2=N&HT=QQ&LCT=LL&FS=S1&FR=R1&FG=G1&FA=A1&FI=I1&FP=P1&FSL=S1&FRL=R1&FGL=G1&FAL=A1&FIL=I1&FPL=P1&PV=&TST=False&C1=&C2=&QP=G&DP=1&VA=CI&CS=Y&SYID=&EYID=&SC=DEFAULT&SO=ASC.

145. https://nccd.cdc.gov/Youthonline/App/Results.aspx-?TT=A&OUT=0&SID=HS&QID=QQ&LID=XX&YID=2017&LID2=&Y-

ID2=&COL=S&ROW1=N&ROW2=N&HT=QQ&LCT=LL&FS=S1&-
FR=R1&FG=G1&FA=A1&FI=I1&FP=P1&FSL=S1&FRL=R1&FGL=G1&-
FAL=A1&FIL=I1&FPL=P1&PV=&TST=False&C1=&C2=&QP=G&D-
P=1&VA=CI&CS=Y&SYID=&EYID=&SC=DEFAULT&SO=ASC.

146. "High School YRBS." *Centers for Disease Control and Prevention*, Centers for Disease Control and Prevention, 2020, nccd.cdc.gov/Youthonline/App/ Default.aspx.

147. Secades-Villa, Roberto, et al. "Probability and predictors of the cannabis gateway effect: a national study." *The International Journal on Drug Policy*, vol. 26,2 (2015): 135-42. DOI: 10.1016/j.drugpo.2014.07.011.

148. Taylor, Michelle, et al. "Patterns of cannabis use during adolescence and their association with harmful substance use behaviour: findings from a UK birth cohort." *Journal of Epidemiology and Community Health*, vol. 71,8 (2017): 764-770. DOI: 10.1136/jech-2016-208503.

149. The National Center on Addiction and Substance Abuse (CASA) at Columbia University. *2011 Family Dinners Report Finds: Teens Who Have Infrequent Family Dinners Likelier to Smoke, Drink, Use Marijuana*, 22 Sept. 2011, www.prnewswire.com/news-releases/2011-family-dinners-report-finds-teens-who-have-infrequent-family-dinners-likelier-to-smoke-drink-use-marijuana-130326838.html.

150. "The Ultimate Do's and Don'ts Guide for Talking to Your Kids about Drug and Alcohol Abuse." *Vertava Health Texas*, 24 Feb. 2021, www.treehouserehab.org/talking-kids-about-drug-alcohol-abuse/.

151. "Talking to Your Child About Drugs (for Parents) - Nemours KidsHealth." Edited by Rupal Christine Gupta, *KidsHealth*, The Nemours Foundation, Nov. 2014, www.kidshealth.org/en/parents/talk-about-drugs.html.

152. The National Center on Addiction and Substance Abuse (CASA) at Columbia University. *2011 Family Dinners Report Finds: Teens Who Have Infrequent Family Dinners Likelier to Smoke, Drink, Use Marijuana*, 22 Sept. 2011, www.prnewswire.com/news-releases/2011-family-dinners-report-finds-teens-who-have-infrequent-family-dinners-likelier-to-smoke-drink-use-marijuana-130326838.html.

153. https://johnnysambassadors.org/thc/.

154. Di Forti, Marta, et al. "Daily use, especially of high-potency cannabis, drives the earlier onset of psychosis in cannabis users." *Schizophrenia Bulletin*, vol. 40,6 (2014): 1509-17. DOI: 10.1093/schbul/sbt181.

155. Hlavinka, Elizabeth. "Meta-Analysis: Even One THC Hit Carries Risk for Inducing Psychosis." *Medical News and Free CME Online*, MedpageTo-

day, 17 Mar. 2020, www.medpagetoday.com/psychiatry/generalpsychia-try/85472.

156. "Drinking Alcohol in Excess Kills Brain Cells." *Scientific American Mind,* vol. 23, no. 2, 16 May 2012, pp. 10–10., DOI: 10.1038/scientificamerican-mind0512-10c.

157. Somerville, Leah H. "The Teenage Brain." *Current Directions in Psychological Science,* vol. 22, no. 2, 2013, pp. 121–127., DOI: 10.1177/0963721413476512.

158. Nourbakhsh, Mahra, et al. "Cannabinoid Hyperemesis Syndrome: Reports of Fatal Cases." *Journal of Forensic Sciences,* vol. 64,1 (2019): 270-274. DOI: 10.1111/1556-4029.13819.

159. Fields, Asia. "Fatal Rainier Valley House Fire Likely Caused by Marijuana Grow Light, Investigators Say." *The Seattle Times,* The Seattle Times Company, 23 Jan. 2019, www.seattletimes.com/seattle-news/fatal-rainier-val-ley-house-fire-likely-caused-by-marijuana-grow-light-investigators-say/.

160. "Fatal Car Accidents Involving Marijuana Have Tripled in U.S." *Hg.org,* Ankin Law Office LLC, www.hg.org/legal-articles/fatal-car-accidents-in-volving-marijuana-have-tripled-in-u-s--32314.

161. "Marijuana 'Dabbing' Causing Explosions and Severe Burns." *Partnership to End Addiction,* 3 Apr. 2017, drugfree.org/drug-and-alcohol-news/mari-juana-dabbing-causing-explosions-severe-burns/.

162. Nourbakhsh, Mahra, et al. "Cannabinoid Hyperemesis Syndrome: Reports of Fatal Cases." *Journal of Forensic Sciences,* vol. 64,1 (2019): 270-274. DOI: 10.1111/1556-4029.13819.

163. Silins, Edmund, et al. "Young Adult Sequelae of Adolescent Cannabis Use: an Integrative Analysis." *The Lancet,* vol. 1, no. 4, Sept. 2014, pp. 286–293., DOI: https://doi.org/10.1016/S2215-0366(14)70307-4.

164. Sund, Reijo, et al. "Substance-Induced Psychoses Converting Into Schizo-phrenia: A Register-Based Study of 18,478 Finnish Inpatient Cases." *Psy-chiatrist.com,* 17 Apr. 2012, www.psychiatrist.com/jcp/schizophrenia/sub-stance-use-disorders/substance-induced-psychoses-converting-schizophrenia/.

165. Starzer, Marie Stefanie, et al. "Rates and Predictors of Conversion to Schizophrenia or Bipolar Disorder Following Substance-Induced Psy-chosis." *American Journal of Psychiatry,* vol. 175, no. 4, 28 Nov. 2017, pp. 343–350., DOI: 10.1176/appi.ajp.2017.17020223.

166. "Key Findings: Recovery: The Many Paths to Wellness." *Key Findings: Recovery: The Many Paths to Wellness | Surgeon General's Report on Al-*

cohol, Drugs, and Health, addiction.surgeongeneral.gov/key-findings/recovery.

167. "Recovery Definitions." *NAADAC - The Association of Addiction Professionals,* www.naadac.org/recovery-definitions.

168. Hodgins, David C., and Jonathan N. Stea. "Insights from Individuals Successfully Recovered from Cannabis Use Disorder: Natural versus Treatment-Assisted Recoveries and Abstinent versus Moderation Outcomes." *Addiction Science & Clinical Practice,* vol. 13, no. 1, 30 July 2018, DOI: 10.1186/s13722-018-0118-0.

169. "The Brain in Recovery." *Recovery Research Institute,* www.recoveryanswers.org/recovery-101/brain-in-recovery/.

170. Gilman, J. M., et al. "Why We Like to Drink: A Functional Magnetic Resonance Imaging Study of the Rewarding and Anxiolytic Effects of Alcohol." *Journal of Neuroscience,* vol. 28, no. 18, 30 Apr. 2008, pp. 4583–4591., DOI: 10.1523/jneurosci.0086-08.2008.

171. Volkow, N.D., et al. "Imaging Dopamine's Role in Drug Abuse and Addiction." *Neuropharmacology,* vol. 56, 2009, pp. 3–8., DOI: 10.1016/j.neuropharm.2008.05.022.

172. Koob, George F. "The Neurobiology of Addiction: a Neuroadaptational View Relevant for Diagnosis." *Society for the Study of Addiction,* vol. 101, 8 Aug. 2006, pp. 23–30., DOI: 10.1111/j.1360-0443.2006.01586.x.

173. Smith, Fran. "How Science Is Unlocking the Secrets of Drug Addiction." *Magazine,* National Geographic, 10 Feb. 2021, www.nationalgeographic.com/magazine/2017/09/the-addicted-brain/.

174. Witkiewitz, Katie, et al. "Retraining the Addicted Brain: A Review of Hypothesized Neurobiological Mechanisms of Mindfulness-Based Relapse Prevention." *Psychology of Addictive Behaviors,* vol. 27, no. 2, 2013, pp. 351–365., DOI: 10.1037/a0029258.

175. Linke, Sarah E., and Michael Ussher. "Exercise-based treatments for substance use disorders: evidence, theory, and practicality." *The American Journal of Drug and Alcohol Abuse,* vol. 41,1 (2015): 7-15. DOI: 10.3109/00952990.2014.976708.

176. Chadi, Nicholas, et al. "Moving beyond perceived riskiness: Marijuana-related beliefs and marijuana use in adolescents." *Substance Abuse,* vol. 41,3 (2020): 297-300. DOI: 10.1080/08897077.2019.1635972.

Made in the USA
Monee, IL
30 April 2024

57769148R00184